Polly Tommey is founder and Editor-in-Chief of the *Autism File* Global and founder of The Autism Trust. She is renowned as a campaigning and influential journalist and is featured regularly as an expert in the national media. **Jonathan Tommey** is a well-respected nutritional practitioner and runs an autism clinic where he has around 700 children in his care.

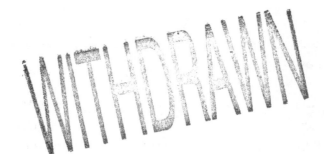

Autism

A practical guide to improving your child's quality of life

JONATHAN TOMMEY and
POLLY TOMMEY

piatkus

PIATKUS

First published in Great Britain in 2011 by Piatkus

A CIP catalogue record for this book
is available from the British Library.

The suggestions and treatments described in this book should not replace
the care and direct supervision of a trained healthcare professional. The
recommendations given in this book are intended solely as education and
information and should not be taken as medical advice. Neither the authors
nor the publisher accept liability for readers who choose to self-prescribe.

ISBN 978-0-7499-4238-0

Typeset in Utopia by Paul Saunders
Printed and bound in Great Britain by MPG Books, Bodmin, Cornwall

Papers used by Piatkus are natural, renewable and recyclable
products sourced from well-managed forests and certified
in accordance with the rules of the Forest Stewardship Council.

Mixed Sources
Product group from well-managed
forests and other controlled sources
www.fsc.org Cert no. SGS-COC-004081
© 1996 Forest Stewardship Council
FSC

Piatkus
An imprint of
Little, Brown Book Group
100 Victoria Embankment
London EC4Y ODY

An Hachette UK Company
www.hachette.co.uk

www.piatkus.co.uk

To Bella, Billy and Toby for living life a little differently than planned. And to Richard Barber, who passionately believed in all of us.

Contents

Acknowledgements

Without the following people Billy would not be where he is today: Barbara Barber, Margaret Barron, Paul Shattock OBE, Rosemary Kessick, Kenneth Bock, Mandi Rodwell, Raj Mann, Carol Stott, Andrew and Carmel Wakefield, Arthur Krigsman, Jim Moody, Stephanie Lord, David O'Connell, Sally Bunday, William Shaw, Michael Ash, Ann Jones, Lisa Galton, Garry Curtis, Dave Humprey, Willis S. Langford, Devin Houston, Natasha Campbell McBride, Bernie Rimland, Teri and Ed Arranga, Julie Matthews, Chantal Sicile-Kira, all the Treating Autism team, Autism One, DAN, NAA, NAI and the CryShame team, Curt and Kim Linderman, Gordon and Sarah Brown, Jan and Alf Percival, Natalie Williams, Alli Edwards, Andrew, Matt and James Tommey, Rosie, Dave and Kitty Baker, Jamie, Ella, Teddy, Louis and Jem Barber, Harriet, Daniel, Dorelia and Maeve Thompson, Wendy, John and Georgia Hinchcliffe, Kathy Barber, Mary and Martin Ganderton, Geoff and Simone Sewell, Belinda and Michael Nunn, Glynis Barber and Michael Brandon, Sally Beck, Caroline Traa, Joan Campbell, John Stone, Isabella Thomas, Heidi, Charlie, Lottie and Oscar Rees, Emma Cope, Liese and Robin Cairns, Sally and David Rowland, Fiona Mayne, Ray, Sarah and Indie Galton, Peter Mead, Jonathan Lewis, Milti and Rachel Christodoulou, Sarah Sherwood, Jackie Doe, Carla Hill, Jon, Fiona and Gregor Sumner, Philip and Liese Ganderton, David Liddiment, Robert and Lucy Dorrien Smith. The islanders of Tresco, Isles of Scilly. Bill Welsh,

Ralph and Patricia Kanter, Sir Anthony Hopkins, Lady Jenni Hopkins, Robert and Sally Greene, Guy and Marrion Naggar, Linda Cooper, Terry O'Neil, Lorraine Ashton, Tony Pinkus, Simon Ranger, Tania Bryer, Eddie and Lisa Villiers, Sue Peart from *You* magazine for believing in the Autism Mothers campaign, Autism Mothers and Fathers worldwide.

Abbreviations Used in the Book

ABA: applied behaviour analysis

ABC: antecedent, behaviour and consequences

ADHD: attention deficit disorder (also attention deficit hyperactivity disorder)

AIA: Allergy Induced Autism

ASC: autism spectrum condition

ASDAN: Award Scheme Development and Accreditation Network

BERIS: body basics, environment, relatedness, insight and self-belief

CARD: Center for Autism and Related Disorders

CDD: childhood disintegrative disorder

CDSA: comprehensive digestive stool analysis

CHAT: CHecklist for Autism in Toddlers

CNS: central nervous system

DAN: Defeat Autism Now

DPT: diphtheria, pertussis and tetanus vaccination

EEG: electroencephalography

EIBI: Early Intensive Behavioural Intervention

ENS: enteric nervous system

ENT: ear, nose and throat

ESPA: Education and Services for People with Autism

FOS: fructo-oligosaccharides

GFCF: gluten-free, casein-free

GI: gastrointestinal

IBS: irritable bowel syndrome

IEP: individual education programme

IIT: intensive interaction therapy

LA: local authority

MMR: measles, mumps and rubella vaccination

MRSA: methicillin-resistant *Staphylococcus aureus*

NAC: N-acetyl cysteine

NET: natural environment training

NVQ: National Vocational Qualification

OT: occupational therapist

PDBE: polybrominated diphenyl ether

PDD-NOS: pervasive developmental disorder – not otherwise specified

PECS: Picture Exchange Communication System

PFOA: perfluorooctanoic acid

SALT: speech and language therapist

SAMe: S-adenosylmethionine

SCD: specific carbohydrate diet

SEN: special educational needs

SENCO: special educational needs coordinator

SEND: Special Educational Needs and Disability

SPD: sensory processing disorder

TEACCH: Treatment and Education of Autistic and related Communication-handicapped Children

TSC: tuberous sclerosis complex

VB: verbal behaviour approach

Introduction

My husband, Jon, and I have three beautiful children. Our second child and eldest son, Billy, was diagnosed with severe autism at two and a half. It changed our lives.

Our desire to find as much information as possible about the condition, its causes and potential treatments, and to do whatever is necessary to improve Billy's life, has led us on an extraordinary journey, and we now live a life dedicated to improving the lives of people with autism everywhere.

Autism, or autism spectrum condition (ASC), describes a range of developmental and behavioural issues arising from a brain that is somehow 'wired up' differently, affecting the way it processes information from the senses and manages the mental connections necessary to develop or use the complex social, language and thinking skills that most people take for granted.

Nobody really knows exactly how or why this happens. It is generally accepted that there is a genetic component, but there could be any number of different ways to activate this genetic potential. Some children show signs right from birth, whereas others, like Billy, seem to develop perfectly normally and then to suddenly regress.

Children with autism will have some level of difficulty with understanding and using language in all its forms, they'll have trouble relating to others, particularly when it comes to interpreting other people's needs, expectations or emotions, and they will have problems with any kind of flexible or abstract thought. Many children will also have sensitivity issues regarding touch, light or sound, and many will develop strange or challenging physical mannerisms and behaviours.

Following Billy's diagnosis in November 1998, and based on our early efforts to gather as much information as possible and to share it as widely as possible, I began publishing a quarterly magazine, the *Autism File* (www.autismfile.com) from home in autumn 1999, to cover all aspects of autism research and information for parents like us. It has now grown into a leading international journal, providing practical guidance and academic research on a wide range of medical, nutritional and educational issues. Through this publication I have been able to connect with thousands of parents all over the world who are living with autism and with the doctors, scientists, therapists and educationalists who are striving to help.

Our subsequent immersion in all things nutritional and biomedical in our efforts to help Billy led Jon to take a second degree, in nutritional therapy, and to set up The Autism Clinic (www.theautismclinic.com). Through the clinic, Jon identifies, supports and treats a range of health and well-being issues affecting many people with autism, applying treatment protocols involving a variety of highly specific dietary, nutritional and therapeutic approaches. He has now seen and helped over 500 children and their families.

More recently, our dismay at learning how potentially bleak the future was for Billy once he left school, and the woeful lack of provision and life-opportunities in general for people with autism as they move through schooling into adulthood, led me to found our charity, The Autism Trust (www.theautismtrust. org.uk), in January 2007. The Trust is dedicated to building sustainable futures for people with autism by setting up Centres of Excellence to provide outstanding, innovative support for the well-being, employment, ongoing education and care of people with autism and their families.

Our journey with Billy and autism has been hard at times and I won't pretend that it is ever an easy ride but if, as a parent of a child with autism, you persevere and stay strong, you will see that it is possible to improve the life of your child. You will feel emotions that you didn't even know you had, you will become part of a community, meeting parents and carers who are some of the strongest, most intelligent people you will ever meet, you will make the best friends you could ever have hoped for – friends for life – and at times you will laugh or cry so hard your body will ache.

The love we all have for our children, whether with autism or not, is endless – love is the most important gift we can ever give.

At times your love will be tested and there will be occasions when you will cry out in desperation, but one thing I know for sure is that this journey will change you for the better and you will, without doubt, burst with pride at your child's every achievement and, because they have to work that little bit harder than a child without autism, every moment will be special.

Please know that you are not alone. As parents of children with autism, we are all in this together – and together we will strive for answers and solutions.

Through 13 years of living and working with autism, we have learned one very valuable lesson: that each and every child with autism is different. So we cannot give you a single solution, there *is* no single solution, but we will show you what worked for Billy and what treatments, therapies, programmes, strategies and approaches are available out there that might help your child.

I have written many articles over the years about Billy's progress and achievements, and the treatment protocols we were implementing at the time. Afterwards, I would get calls and emails from parents saying that their own child was 'identical' to Billy, so they would rigidly follow Billy's therapy or supplement regime. Of course, no two children are identical, so some did but some didn't get similar results.

Children may share similar traits and behaviours, but they will be different inside. They will have a different physiological make-up, with different allergies, different biomedical problems, different medical histories and different genes! So although Billy might do well with a certain therapy, it may have absolutely no effect on another child, and vice versa. This is a vitally important starting point when reading anything on autism. We wasted too many years soldiering on with a therapy just because it worked for another child, and assuming it must work for Billy. But we also learned a lot from the experiences of others, and helped Billy by trying what the other parents tried.

The main advice we can give anyone is to read, listen and learn but, as parents, ultimately you will know your child better than anyone else; for example, if you start a therapy or treatment and your 'gut' feeling is that it is not right, then trust yourself and stop it or change it. Having said that, you will also come to know when to 'push on' for the treatment to work – it's a fine line.

We have made many mistakes on our autism journey – most of us do; however, the only way to deal with your mistakes is to pick yourself up, brush them aside, learn and move on. We have also done an awful lot right!

We have come a long way from the day when I went to the library, pulled out a book and looked up 'autism'. All I can remember of that dark day is the words, 'The most severe form of mental illness, there is no cure; most if not all will be institutionalised.' We now know that this is simply not the case. We know so much more now; there is a great deal that can be done to improve the quality of life for people with autism.

Billy's autism was initially severe: he lived in his own world, he banged his head and screamed most of the time, his hair fell out and he lost all speech and communication from the age of 13 to 18 months. Billy had major health issues. He is now 14 years old and is described as 'high functioning'. He can speak, read and write and, although Billy still has autism, never in my wildest dreams did I expect him to progress as he has.

In this book I will take you through our journey and share with you all we have learned through being parents of a child with autism: the successes and setbacks along the way, the knowledge and experience we have gained from living and working with Billy – from those terrible early days to our lives today – from me establishing and editing the *Autism File* and founding The Autism Trust, and from Jon's work in setting up and running The Autism Clinic.

I will share with you everything I have lived through and learned about having a child with autism and Jon will guide you through the scientific and biomedical factors that influence the health, well-being and overall development of your child.

We will look at everything that we know, including therapies and treatments, health and well-being, education and schooling, diet and nutrition, family life and anything else we can think of. We'll take you through the relevant science, the difficult choices and the emotional rollercoaster.

Our aim in sharing our experiences is to help you on your own journey; furnished with as much information as possible about what is happening with your child, what you could try to do about it and where to go to for help. Just be assured that it is possible to improve your child's quality of life. We've done it and you can too.

On this journey we have met and spoken to thousands of parents, teachers, therapists, doctors, scientists and practition-ers worldwide, many of whom have taught us so much, and some of whom will strive to help with all the issues we will tackle in this book. To all of them, many, many thanks.

Polly Tommey

Autism: A Definition

Autism is referred to as a 'spectrum' condition because the specific characteristics may be present in a range of different combinations, which could result from any number of overlapping genetic or developmental disorders. It's also called a 'continuum' because it is possible to have a (relatively) mild or severe form of the condition (or anywhere in between).

The most helpful definition of the core areas of difficulty faced by people with an ASC was described by Lorna Wing and Judy Gould in 1979 as the 'triad of impairments'. Any diagnosis of an ASC will be based on the observation of significant behavioural issues across all three areas, with a continuum of need and severity within each as described briefly below:

Impairment of social interaction includes fundamental problems with initiating, understanding or developing personal relationships, from cooperation and turn-taking, through a lack of recognised social skills to a deficiency in the social empathy required to make friends or to comprehend the complex demands of situations that involve an understanding of other people's needs and expectations, or asserting their own.

Impairment of social communication – the 'social' part is important here. It's not just about speech, articulation or vocabulary; it's also about how language is used to communicate with others.

Difficulties might range from a complete absence of functional language, through bizarre, repetitive or pedantic patterns of speech to a lack of understanding of the social nuances of language, such as humour, metaphor, sarcasm, irony or diplomacy.

Impairment of imagination. Often represented as rigidity or inflexibility of thought and lack of pretend play, the full implications of this impairment are often manifested as fundamental problems in 'bringing to mind' or comprehending things that are not immediately accessible via the senses, including unspoken rules, routines or instructions, or abstract thought processes such as anticipating events or outcomes, pretending, adapting to change or planning.

Children with these difficulties may also develop repetitive and stereotyped patterns of behaviour, which could mean, for instance, insisting on always taking the same route, sitting in the same chair or needing to touch every surface, and might involve collecting, arranging or lining up objects, or obsessively sticking to the same limited interests and activities. There might also be elaborate routines or physical mannerisms.

PART 1

FINDING
THE ANSWERS

CHAPTER 1

The First Year

For many of you picking up this book, the first year may not seem particularly relevant, as you will probably already have your child's ASC diagnosis, and this tends to happen in the second or third year (depending on where you live and whether you can afford a private diagnosis). So you're probably already well down the line. But if you're picking up this book because you want to spot the signs or avoid the pitfalls early, or if you are thinking of having another child, then this chapter will help you to avoid the mistakes we made with Billy as, with the benefit of hindsight, we realise that they were crucial.

Jon and I have two boys, Billy and Toby. Both, we believe, were born healthy and with no obvious problems; however, our boys had very different first years and I am going to set out for you the things we did and those we wish we had or hadn't done.

This pivotal part of the story centres on some of the key features of Billy's infancy, particularly breastfeeding, weaning, childhood infections and antibiotics.

Early days

Billy was born a healthy 3.74kg (8lb 4oz) on 30 April 1996, 16 months after his sister, Bella. He was delivered in a different hospital from Bella so I had a different midwife. We were told she was excellent and we couldn't be in better hands. I had met this midwife before as she had visited us at home when I was struggling with breastfeeding Bella. She remembered that visit and, as soon as Billy was born, she handed me a bottle of formula feed. 'It's better this way,' she said in a matronly manner. 'You struggled with your daughter. Sometimes it's easier to do it this way … I've been a midwife for thirty years!'

As our story unfolds, you will see that I have met many so-called 'experts' along the way, and it is through following these people's advice that I have probably made my biggest mistakes. In this case, the midwife was certainly experienced, but my gut feeling would have been to at least try to breastfeed Billy. But she was the 'expert'. I put my faith in her experience and I bowed to her advice.

Billy was subsequently deprived of the benefits of breastfeeding and was bottle-fed with formula right from the start. We now see this as a critical error in Billy's case. Breast milk is a live, organic and natural food that is specifically 'designed' to match your baby's nutritional needs, whereas the developing immune system of some babies reacts in an allergic way to cow's milk protein. It is also worth noting that cow's milk protein taken in by a nursing mother is passed to the baby in her breast milk. This can be a source of allergy and, if so, the mother may need to exclude cow's milk from her own diet.

The benefits of breastfeeding

Breastfeeding is a natural process, which is important for babies and for mums. Breast milk is the ideal food for babies. It contains the right combination of proteins, fats, carbohydrates, vitamins, minerals, fluids and antibodies to nourish your baby and to protect it against infection while its own natural defences develop.

Breastfeeding your baby from day one until at least six months, and preferably until one year, has been shown to deliver a wide range of specific health benefits in the short, medium and long term; for example, immediate benefits to your baby's health and development, and better health through life.

Unfortunately, breastfeeding doesn't work for everyone. This might be due to any number of reasons, from medical issues to lifestyle choices. Many women who want to breast-feed find that they (or their baby) simply can't for one reason or another, and many women who could, find that bottle-feeding suits them better, particularly if they need to return to work relatively soon after the birth of their baby. (I give some suggestions for alternatives on pages 19–20.)

Following the advice I had from the midwife, my little Billy started his life on cow's milk formula – drinking gallons of it; indeed, he couldn't get enough but, despite his ravenous appetite, things were going pretty much to plan. He had all his DPT (diphtheria, pertussis and tetanus) jabs and boosters according to schedule at two, three and four months and seemed to be thriving. By the time he was five months old he was sucking so hard that the teat would get vacuumed back into the bottle. We had no choice but to put him on a feeder cup. He still sucked it dry, although he would often throw up immediately afterwards, and would get bright red ears (which we now know is a common response to food allergies). It was at this point that I was advised by a medical friend to put Billy on pasteurised cow's milk, straight from the carton but slightly warmed – he loved it. This was another huge mistake.

The health visitor came to visit us when Billy was five months old and she suggested that because Billy was always so desper-ately hungry, we should start solids early. I gave him breadsticks to chew on; he carried them everywhere and gorged himself on them.

I now know that starting Billy on breadsticks at five months certainly wasn't a good idea; in fact, most health experts expressly warn against the early introduction of foods containing wheat and gluten, as a baby's digestive and immune systems are still developing, and these foods can cause allergies. For the same reason, it's not advisable to give them foods containing eggs, fish, shellfish, nuts, seeds and soft or unpasteurised cheese at any time before six months. Cow's milk is also a bad idea as a main drink before 12 months, as it doesn't have enough iron or vitamins C and D. (Not to mention that babies are not calves, so I'm struggling to understand why we are recommended to use cow's milk in the first place.)

My health visitor gave me no advice on this, so I had no idea that the foods I was giving Billy were doing him no good.

Coughs and infections

Billy was more than content with his cow's milk cup and his breadsticks, and was a happy, chubby five-month-old when suddenly he developed a nasty cough. I rushed him to the doctor, who immediately prescribed Billy's first dose of antibiotics: amoxicillin, a broad-spectrum antibiotic from the penicillin group (see page 8). The cough didn't get better and seemed to set in, and it was closely followed by an ear infection. Over the next few months he was plagued by recurrent chest and ear infections and was back and forth to the doctor.

In his first year of life, Billy had six courses of antibiotics for chest and ear infections. When the doctor told me to come back if Billy didn't get better, I did. His courses alternated between amoxicillin, cephalexin and erythromycin, but the cough and the ear infections just stayed the same.

Toby, Billy's younger brother, also suffered from recurrent chesty cough and ear infections after five months but, because of what we had learned with Billy, he's never had a course of antibiotics. As I write, he is a fit and healthy 12-year-old who has never even been to the doctor!

The difference so far between the two boys, is that Toby was brought up on rice milk formula and then rice milk, with no casein or gluten in the first two years, and with illnesses treated with homeopathy. When Toby was really ill with a chesty cough and high temperature we put cold flannels on his forehead to lower his temperature and dosed him with homeopathic remedies. The point here is that neither of the boys needed antibiotics, but Billy was completely saturated with them. Antibiotics obviously have their place, but should only be used sparingly, and only when they are absolutely necessary.

What is homeopathy?

Homeopathy is a type of alternative medicine that uses highly diluted substances, usually from plants and minerals, to trigger the body's own natural defences and healing processes. It is based on the concept that substances that cause symptoms in otherwise healthy people, which match the symptoms experienced by the patient, could, in infinitesimally small quantities, prompt the patient's body to recognise the culprit and use its innate 'vital energy' to heal itself.

As part of Jon's research into the causes of autism, he asked families who had a child with autism to complete a questionnaire detailing their own and their child's medical history. One key finding was the large proportion of children with autism (68 per cent of responses) who had received multiple courses of antibiotics in their first year.

Antibiotics

I need to tell you a little about antibiotics and the effects they can have on the digestive system and the immune systems. (Jon will explain about the gut, the immune system and their relationship to autism later in the book.)

Antibiotics are powerful drugs that are used to treat disease and infection by killing or neutralising bacteria. The first antibiotic, penicillin, was discovered by accident in 1928, when the scientist Alexander Fleming realised that the mould (fungus) that had grown on the cultures of bacteria he was studying in his lab had killed the bacteria. Antibiotics didn't become available as medicines until the Second World War, but there are now over 100 different types available and they are the most frequently prescribed drugs in modern medicine. In 2008, general practitioners in Britain wrote 38 million prescriptions for them.

What can be treated with antibiotics?

Although antibiotics are used to treat a variety of infections, it is important to note that they can only be effective against bacterial infections (such as strep throat, salmonella, E-coli, and so on) and are useless against viral infections (such as measles, chickenpox and influenza) or fungal and parasitic infections (such as candidiasis – yeast infection – athlete's foot or ringworm). Unfortunately, many people (and indeed doctors) just aren't aware of this and expect, or even demand, antibiotics for all sorts of illnesses that they would be completely ineffective at treating.

Some antibiotics are only effective against particular species of bacteria, whereas others, the broad-spectrum antibiotics, attack a wide range of bacteria. Many of the most familiar and most commonly prescribed antibiotics (such as amoxicillin) fall into the second category.

What's wrong with broad-spectrum antibiotics?

Although broad-spectrum might seem like a good thing, it is often quite the reverse, as these types of antibiotics do not distinguish between the harmful bacteria that are causing the infection and the beneficial bacteria that live in our gut and perform a huge range of vital functions in the digestive and immune systems.

The antibiotic problem

We must not forget that antibiotics, when used specifically to treat known bacterial infections, are a precious resource whose benefits can certainly outweigh their risks. They can often be the only effective treatment for life-threatening infections and diseases; however, we are aware that some doctors tend to over-prescribe antibiotics for comparatively minor infections, often under the pressure of caring parents or due to over-caution, and may apply them without first testing to identify the specific type of infection. This can have a devastating effect on the body's natural defences, especially as the overuse of antibiotics can also lead to various species of bacteria becoming resistant to the effects of the very antibiotics sent in to attack them. Those bacteria that are naturally stronger or more resistant tend to reproduce, creating colonies of resistant strains.

The normal functioning of the intestinal tract (the gut) depends upon the presence of huge numbers of hundreds of species of beneficial bacteria, known collectively as the gut flora. There are ten times more bacteria in the gut than there are cells in the human body, typically between 3kg (6lb 8oz) and 3.5kg (7¾lb) in an adult! These vast and complex colonies of microorganisms exist in a symbiotic relationship with humans (living together in mutually beneficial harmony). We keep them fed and they serve a vital purpose in the digestion of food and in supporting the body's immune system, keeping us healthy by coating and defending every surface of the gut wall, suppressing or warding off harmful bacteria as well as fungal, parasitic and viral pathogens (microbes that cause illness and disease) and toxins, and preventing them from spreading or penetrating the gut wall to cause infection or disease.

Why gut flora are so important

Gut flora play a vital role in the digestion and absorption of food and nutrients by fermenting soluble fibre, and synthesising (building from component parts) short-chain fatty acids and vitamins, both of which are essential for breaking down food and extracting nutrients and energy. They help to produce the body's most active and effective antioxidant, glutathione (more on antioxidants later), and are instrumental in the production of vitamin K (needed for blood-clotting and healing) and a whole range of B vitamins, notably biotin, which is necessary for the process of extracting energy from food, and B_{12} which is vital for the production of red blood cells and for the metabolism of every cell in the body. They also stimulate the production of antibodies (known as immunoglobulins) such as the hugely important secretory IgA (sec IgA), the neurotransmitter serotonin and chemical messengers called cytokines.

Antibodies act as agents of the immune system to seek out and destroy harmful bacteria, parasites, viruses and fungi. IgA is the main antibody that protects the lining of the gut (mucosa) from infection by these pathogens. Serotonin supports peristalsis – the muscular contractions of the gut that move food through the system – and is vital as a neurotransmitter in the brain to regulate mood, appetite, sleep and some cognitive functions such as memory and learning. Cytokines carry messages to the immune system to tell them which harmful microbes to attack and which antibodies are needed for the job. One of these cytokines – gamma interferon – is one of the body's most effective, front-line defences against viral infections, fungal infections and tumours.

Our understanding of the complex role of the gut flora is still in its infancy, but the more we discover, the more it becomes clear just how vital they are to our health and well-being. So much so that many people consider the gut flora to be 'the forgotten organ'.

What happens when gut flora are destroyed?

The actions of broad-spectrum antibiotics, in wiping out huge numbers of beneficial bacteria along with the harmful ones among the gut flora, can therefore result in significant deficiencies in vitamin K, B vitamins, glutathione, serotonin, short-chain fatty acids, immunoglobulins and cytokines, and so on, and therefore to seriously impair the body's ability to nourish, protect and repair itself.

This disturbance in the delicate balance of beneficial and potentially harmful microorganisms in the gut is known as dysbiosis, which is, quite literally, the opposite of the symbiosis that normally characterises the relationship of the gut flora to the host (us).

If the beneficial bacteria aren't present in sufficient numbers to keep pathogens in check, and the lining of the gut has lost some of its immune protection, it is in a state of dysbiosis, and these pathogens can start to spread, seizing on the opportunity to colonise, attacking defenceless cells, including those in the lining of the gut wall itself (the mucosa), and causing so-called 'opportunistic infections'. Two of the most common side effects of taking antibiotics are the diarrhoea and colitis (inflammation of the colon), caused by the bacterium *Clostridium difficile* and the yeast infection candidiasis caused by the yeast *Candida albicans*. Both of these are often present in the gut, but are normally dominated and suppressed by good bacteria.

Once these pathogenic bacteria and others like them begin to spread, they can colonise large areas of the gut, where they not only cause infections and damage other cells but they also start to process and digest food in a different way, consuming nutrients rather than passing them on, and producing toxins (such as proprionic acid) instead of beneficial vitamins and short-chain fatty acids, and so on, leaving the host deficient and malnourished.

The damage to the lining of the gut wall can be severe enough to make it more permeable (easier to penetrate), allowing larger molecules from food residue to leak through the gut wall into the bloodstream before they are properly digested. This causes allergic reactions and allows pathogens and toxins into the bloodstream – a condition we've come to know as 'leaky gut'. Significant examples of the larger molecules allowed to leak through the gut wall under these circumstances are the un-digested proteins from gluten and casein that contribute to negative reactions to dairy and wheat products.

About gluten and casein

Gluten is a combination of two proteins (gliadin and glu-tanin) found in wheat and a number of other cereals (rye, barley, bulgur, durum, kamut and spelt). Oats are also often avoided by people on a gluten-free, casein-free (GFCF) diet due to a gluten-like protein and to the high risk of contamination with other cereals during processing. Gluten and/or similar proteins are also found in semolina, couscous, malt, soy sauce and in some colourings and flavourings.

Casein is the predominant protein found in cow's milk and dairy products (such as cheese, butter, cream, yoghurt and ice cream). It is particularly concentrated in cheese. Casein also crops up in the form of an added ingredient, caseinate, in some non-dairy products such as soya cheese.

When not properly digested, these proteins form the opioid peptides gluteomorphin and casomorphin, which can have an affect on brain functioning similar to the effects of morphine, causing damage to the parts of the brain that control learning, attention and communication.

In addition to its detrimental effects on the immune system (called immunosuppression) and the development of resistant bacterial species, the overuse of antibiotics (particularly multiple courses of broad-spectrum antibiotics) can also cause a range of serious medical conditions such as leucopoenia (a reduction in the production of white blood cells, increasing the risk of infection), pancreatitis (inflammation of the pancreas, causing acute abdominal pain and impaired digestion), hyperkalemia (elevated levels of potassium in the blood, leading to the risk of arrhythmia – abnormal heart rhythm), chronic diarrhoea, eczema and other skin rashes.

Interestingly, and somewhat ironically, the bacteria that Alexander Fleming was studying when he discovered the antibacterial effects of penicillin were the *Staphylococcus* bacteria. A strain of this very bacterium is the potentially lethal culprit at the heart of the so-called 'superbug', MRSA. MRSA stands for methicillin-resistant *Staphylococcus aureus*; in other words, the bacteria have developed a resistance to methicillin, a narrow-spectrum antibiotic in the penicillin class, as well as to penicillin itself, and to another popular penicillin derivative, amoxicillin.

Does this mean that antibiotics are immunosuppressant drugs?

Although it is clear that this is not the intention of prescribing antibiotics, and that their primary action is to kill infectious bacteria, it is also clear that they do have a suppressing effect on our ability to maintain our own natural defences against infection by disrupting the balance of the gut flora and of resident bacteria on all the body's mucous membranes.

The specific effect of antibiotics on the immune system depends on the general state of health of the individual, the type of antibiotic and the strength and length of the course. Babies, small children, old people and those who are generally weak and

ill are at greatest risk, as they are naturally more prone to infection, have weaker immune systems and are more likely to be
prescribed antibiotics.

Back in 1972, Professor Sandy Raeburn, Head of the Department of Clinical Genetics at Nottingham University and a
specialist in diseases of young children, wrote: 'Immunological
deficiency syndromes were not observed before 1952. A possible
explanation is some of these conditions are produced by the
administration of antibiotics to certain individuals at a critical
point in the development of immune responses.'

Dr Raeburn observed that 'antibiotics should be reserved
for life-threatening infections until the risk of immunotoxicity
is excluded in each patient, especially if the patient is immunosuppressed.'

The immune systems of children with autism

Did multiple courses of broad-spectrum antibiotics, prescribed
for early mucosal infections in our children who have autism
suppress their immune systems?

Children with autism seem particularly susceptible to mucosal infections; for example, in the nose, ears and respiratory
system. Infections in all these areas are common in young
children, and particularly in children with an ASC diagnosis.
They include various gastrointestinal infections, diarrhoea or
constipation, bronchitis (chest infection), rhinitis (runny nose)
and otitis media (ear infections and glue ear).

None of Billy's various courses of antibiotics managed to clear
up the infections, and there is a strong probability that their use
left him severely immunosuppressed and unable to cope with the
pathogenic onslaught delivered by antibiotic-resistant and/or
opportunistic bacteria, yeast species and parasitic infections.

He certainly had an overgrowth of the bacterium *Clostridium
difficile*, plus parasites and candidiasis of the bowel – evidence of
pathogens that are widespread in children with autism.

These issues are becoming increasingly widely known and, as I write this, the European Centre for Disease Control has written to all general practitioners urging them to stop prescribing antibiotics for minor ailments because their widespread and frivolous use is rapidly increasing the number of bacteria that are becoming resistant.

Life for Billy towards the end of his first year

Billy sailed through his hearing test and nine-month check, and then at about ten months he started to babble 'mama' 'dada' 'dis', but he was not in great health, with his constant runny nose, chesty cough and projectile vomiting. (We realised later, that this was not surprising considering the amount of cow's milk and breadsticks he was getting through.)

At 11 months Billy got a nasty case of chickenpox (as did Bella at the same time), so had horrible itching to contend with on top of everything else. It's a common virus that's unpleasant at the best of times, but can be much worse on top of an already weakened system, and Billy had a bad case.

At exactly 12 months old, I took Billy for his MMR vaccination. He still had a chesty cough and a cold, and was still on antibiotics for an ear infection, but this had become the norm with him by then. I let the nurse know that he wasn't well, and she could see it for herself, so advised me to come back in a month's time. She also told me to be careful not to miss this vaccination as 'children like Billy who suffer from ear infections can burst an eardrum or even go deaf if they catch measles'. I wasn't about to let that happen.

Exactly one month later to the day, when Billy was 13 months old, he had the MMR jab.

Considering Billy's general poor health and clearly deficient immune system, and with the benefit of hindsight, we see this as possibly the biggest mistake.

If your baby is unwell when vaccination is due and has only recently finished a course of antibiotics, or has had multiple courses over the previous months, this may have compromised his or her immune system.

It is not my intention to perpetuate the idea that MMR causes autism; however, I do feel that more dedicated independent research is necessary in this area. Research that can be taken further without doctors fearing that their medical licences will be taken away if they speak of their findings. A safe vaccination schedule is all I am asking for.

The chain of events

There are potential genetic factors that may have predisposed Billy to a specifically impaired immune system, including a family history of atopic immune disorders, autoimmune diseases and Th2 dominance (we'll explain this later):

1. Billy's immune system development was compromised by being deprived of the initial benefits of colostrum and the further benefits of breastfeeding.

2. His intake of cow's milk formula led to increased mucus production and either to an allergic reaction created by antigens to the bovine products arising from his under-developed immune system or caused a reaction owing to a genetic intolerance.

3. His compromised immune system allowed the overgrowth in his gut of pathogens such as *Candida* and *Clostridium* species, leading to recurrent mucosal infections, exacerbated by his cow's milk formula consumption and intolerance.

4. The DPT combined vaccine may have presented an early initial insult to his weakened immune system, introducing pathogens and impairing his ability to fight off other, opportunistic pathogens, resulting in their colonisation of

his gut and leading to recurrent respiratory tract and ear infections.

5. Multiple courses of antibiotics administered to counteract the recurrent infections acted upon an already weakened immune system, further depleting beneficial gut flora.

6. This finally caused a state of gut dysbiosis, weakening his immune system still further and possibly resulting in increased gut-wall permeability and the leakage of unmetabolised milk and wheat proteins into his bloodstream.

7. Early transition to full-fat cow's milk and to wheat-based solids exacerbated the implications of existing allergies or intolerances.

8. Contracting the viral infection, chickenpox, while already immunosuppressed and suffering the effects of recurrent infections, weakened Billy's natural defences yet further.

9. The final insult to his immune system of the multiple live virus vaccine, before his system had had time to recover and rebuild, was just too much to handle.

Summary

Autism is increasingly recognised as a genetically predisposed condition that can be triggered by various environmental factors or combinations of circumstances. You've just read about our own situation, but there may be a trillion different routes. Of course, no one is exactly sure what these factors are, but it seems highly likely that they are connected to environmental pollutants, pharmaceutical insults, dietary issues and/or whatever bio-chemical mechanisms underlie the range of gastrointestinal and immunological disorders which seem to go hand in hand with a diagnosis of autism, and particularly with regressive autism.

The most important nuance here is that if autism can be triggered, it can also remain untriggered; if it is not inevitable, then there may be things we can do to minimise the risks and to give our babies the best possible start in life. We can only do what we can, and life is packed with variables, exceptions and unavoidable practicalities, but we suggest you take what you can from our experiences.

How you can help your baby

Here is a summary of our advice for pregnancy and the first year of your baby's life:

During pregnancy and before:

1. If you're thinking of becoming pregnant, it makes sense to ensure that your body is as healthy as possible. Now's the time to detox (*not* once you're pregnant) and to start watching what you eat.

2. There's increasing evidence that molecular changes to your DNA can be caused by your own exposure to drugs, toxins and pollutants, and it's absolutely clear that your baby's immune-system development is dependent on the balance of your own.

3. Consider switching to an organic and hormone-free diet as far as possible and try to use hypo-allergenic cosmetics and household cleaning products. Switch to fluoride-free toothpaste, an aluminium-free deodorant and avoid cooking utensils that are plastic, Teflon-coated or aluminium.

4. Avoid any fish that are even considered moderately high in mercury (you will find a list on page 100). Even the government advises you not to eat certain fish during pregnancy due to its mercury contamination, so it's well worth the sacrifice. Try to avoid plastic packaging and microwave cooking whenever possible right through pregnancy, so choose the loose veg in the supermarket and cook it in the steamer!

5. Make sure you are as healthy as possible through pregnancy: eat a healthy, balanced diet, drink green tea and filtered water and avoid things that might adversely affect your own health and equilibrium – like drinking, smoking, amalgam dental work, taking antibiotics or any other drugs (as far as is safe and possible) and too much fast food. It all has repercussions.

6. Cook only with cold-pressed virgin olive oil and try to leave out any and all saturated or hydrogenated fats (butter, cheap cooking oils, crisps, chips, and so on).

7. Keep your stress levels down and relax as much as possible: get plenty of fresh air and regular massages. Remember that stress isn't just psychological, it's chemical, and cortisol (stress hormone) interacts and interferes with all sorts of metabolic processes.

8. Don't engage in rigorous exercise programmes or saunas.

After the birth:

1. Always question what you're told by 'experts' and put your foot down if you feel strongly about any issue or if you don't feel you have all the objective information you need to make an informed decision. This is your baby, your child.

2. It is important to respect the expertise and experience of others, but you can never afford to do this blindly, and you need to take control of your child's life.

3. Make space in your life for breastfeeding, if you possibly can. Its benefits go way beyond issues of convenience or lifestyle and they can make a huge difference to your baby's (and your own) immediate and life-long health and well-being.

4. At the very least, try to give your baby the benefit of the concentrated nutrients, antibodies and the immune-system start-up kit that is the colostrum you produce over the first three to five days.

5. If breastfeeding is not for you, for whatever reason, the next best thing is to express your breast milk and give that to your baby by bottle. Even if it's in small amounts, it will deliver at least some of its extraordinary benefits. Invest in glass feeding bottles (see page 101 on the problems with plastics) and warm the milk in a pan, not in the microwave.

6. If you're concerned about your own health and diet while breastfeeding, consider further vitamin and mineral supplements, particularly if you're a vegan or if you're not in great health yourself; if you fit either of these categories (or even if you don't) you might want to consult your doctor or a registered nutritionist.

7. If you (or your baby) simply can't breastfeed, then don't despair, but seek out the best formula milk you can find. There are good alternatives to cow's milk formula available, such as Nanny Goat, Neocate and Nutramigen, which are both also hypo-allergenic.

8. Ordinary cow's milk is simply not suitable for any child under six months as it doesn't contain enough of the right fats or vitamins to sustain your baby, and contains far too much sodium and protein.

9. Most medical authorities advise breastfeeding (or formula feeding where necessary) for the first year at least, weaning your baby on to solids (alongside milk) from about six months.

10. Don't make bread (wheat) your baby's first solid food! Use fruit purées and rice cereal instead. Do not introduce eggs, nuts, meat and other grains such as barley, oats and rye until the infant is nine months old.

11. Try to stick to completely natural-fibre baby-wear and bed-linen.

12. Treat your baby's infections as par for the course as much as possible, and do what you can to alleviate the symptoms.

Most infections will sort themselves out within a few days because of your baby's developing natural defences, particularly if you've been able to adhere to the previous advice. Of course, you must visit the doctor as soon as anything worries you, but avoid antibiotics unless you and your doctor are sure that they're absolutely necessary. Ask questions!

CHAPTER 2

Getting a Diagnosis

On the evening of his MMR jab, Billy, at exactly 13 months, developed a high fever, so we dosed him with Calpol and put him to bed. That evening I went to check on him and found him shaking and shivering uncontrollably in his cot. He seemed cold and there was clearly something very wrong, so I wrapped him up snugly, hurriedly got my sister in to babysit for Bella, and Jon and I dashed Billy to the hospital.

The hospital doctor told us, 'He needs a massive course of antibiotics, he's probably had a reaction to the jab; it's quite common.' He also told us that wrapping Billy up warmly had been the wrong thing to do and that we should have stripped him off and let him cool down.

Our little Billy sat on the examination table shivering, his teeth were chattering but his cheeks, tummy, upper arms and legs were bright blotchy red. A different doctor came in and jabbed our 13-month-old with yet another load of antibiotics, telling us that if he hadn't recovered in 48 hours, we should take him back to the doctor.

Two days later, Billy was still feverish and decidedly sick so, as advised, we did take him back to the doctor, who prescribed yet another course of antibiotics; this time a six-week course, to 'really blast everything out', as the doctor put it.

When I look back now I can hardly believe I went along with all these powerful drugs. I was brought up on nettle soup and homeopathy – why was I allowing these doctors to fill my son with all this? My boy was sick, I wanted to do everything right for him, and the doctors knew best – or so I thought.

The decline in Billy's health

Billy deteriorated fast over the next week or so. He lost all his baby speech and began to reject all the foods he'd been happily munching for months. He would eat only wheat biscuits, apples and his beloved milk and breadsticks. He was projectile vomiting after having his antibiotic dose, he would bang his head repeatedly against the back of his chair and let out this extraordinary high-pitched scream. It was unbearable. The worst thing – if there can be anything worse – was the diarrhoea: constant liquid diarrhoea that would seep through every nappy and every piece of clothing. His tummy swelled up, his hair started to fall out and he was losing weight at an alarming rate.

After a few weeks of this, we took him back to the doctor again. We told him everything we could about what was happening with Billy, the change in behaviour and diet, the screaming, and particularly the diarrhoea, and he surmised that the apples were to blame. 'He eats too many apples,' he said, 'don't worry; it's just toddler diarrhoea, he'll grow out of it. Keep him hydrated.'

I did exactly that, though there seemed no shortage of liquids; he was still drinking gallons of milk every day, but nothing changed for the better. The screaming and the head-banging continued day and night for months on end. He became obsessed with the washing machine, lined up objects and watched *Spot the Dog* videos constantly. He became completely withdrawn and simply ignored us all. It was as if Jon and Bella and I just weren't there any more.

Bella was three and as demanding as a three-year-old is supposed to be, I was pregnant again with Toby, and Billy was a constant worry. He screamed and head-banged all day and all night, and Jon and I cried ourselves to sleep listening to him and wondering what on earth had gone so wrong.

We were living close to the end of our tether and Billy's ear infections were still a recurrent issue, so when Jon's dad (a general practitioner from the US) suggested that deafness might be at the root of Billy's problems, we whisked him straight to an ENT specialist.

The specialist told us that Billy would need 'grommets' to fix his glue ear and we were back a month later to have the operation. We were told by the nurse that if he didn't have it, his eardrums were likely to burst. It really was not a happy experience. Billy fought against the anaesthetic and had to be held, literally kicking and screaming, before they could get him to go under.

After the operation, they told us that Billy had had enlarged adenoids and that they'd taken those out as well. To say I was annoyed would be an understatement, as no one had sought my permission for this, or even explained why it was necessary.

Ear infections and glue ear

Middle ear infections are very common in small children who go on to develop autism. In their first year many children develop common viral or bacterial infections or allergies to milk, which can cause inflammation and the production of mucus that blocks the inner ear causing an ear infection. This is called chronic otitis media or glue ear. It may become so inflamed and blocked that grommets need to be inserted into the ear to enable the inner ear to drain.

The 18-month check

At 18 months, our health visitor came to do a routine check on Billy. In the past five months, Billy had regressed severely. Jon and I knew something was very wrong, but we had no idea what it could be. As part of the check, Billy was asked to brush a doll's hair, hand a cup to the health visitor when asked, bang two bricks together, point to his nose and turn to the sound of his name. He couldn't do any of it and, worse still, he appeared to have absolutely no idea what was being asked of him.

The health visitor was clearly concerned. She looked through Billy's records and remarked how well he had done on his nine-month check, when he had passed his challenges easily. Nonetheless, she said he was showing 'strong signs of autism'. This was the first time I had ever heard the word.

I remember immediately going numb, the health visitor mumbled something about making a referral and left, telling me not to worry. Billy was already back watching *Spot the Dog* and it was time to pick Bella up from nursery. I scooped Billy up screaming and shouting. (He always did this when his video was interrupted. I learned to hold him in a special way that meant I wouldn't get head butted by him arching his back and slamming his head against mine.)

Driving to the nursery, listening to Billy's screams, all I could think about was how I was going to tell Jon. Not long after I had met Jon, I remember him telling me that he wanted a son. Not just a son, but a son called Billy. He had always loved that name, he then told me about all the things he wanted for his Billy, the things they'd do together, the cricket, football and rugby games he would take him to. Jon wanted to be the dad he felt he never had. Somehow I felt responsible for Billy not being OK. I couldn't help it, but I felt as though I had let Jon down.

I parked outside the nursery, realised I had a few minutes and took Billy to the park opposite. I watched my son run and run, he didn't once look back or even acknowledge I was there with him.

The long road to diagnosis

It took a year after that, and the whole rigmarole of doctors and psychologists and appointments and assessments and frustrations, to get Billy formally diagnosed, but eventually we got it:

'Severe autism with severe speech and language delay and severe behavioural problems.'

We were lucky – many parents wait a lot longer than that.

The process of diagnosis and the lead up to it can be a lengthy, complex, distressing and frustrating business but will be different for everyone. A lot depends on where you live and on the individual professionals, teams, agencies and personalities involved. Some health authorities and education authorities are better than others at giving help and support through the process, and some even offer specialist nursery places or interventions while a full assessment is undertaken. There are various private options as well, of course, if you can afford it and know where to look.

Without a doubt, we now know that the earlier you can get help, both biomedically and behaviourally, the better. We wasted too many years not doing either, simply because we didn't know. We didn't know we could help Billy, let alone how, and we've had to forge our own path through tiers of health and education professionals and bureaucrats but, that said, we've worked hard with the time we've had, we've learned a huge amount, we've given a huge amount and the results have been incredible.

Understanding the diagnosis

Dr Carol Stott is Scientific Editor of the *Autism File* magazine. She is a chartered psychologist and chartered scientist with the British Psychological Society and has helped us here with the diagnosis procedure.

In most cases, your health visitor or general practitioner will conduct a short questionnaire/screening test as part of your child's routine 18-month check-up. This is called the CHAT (CHecklist for Autism in Toddlers) and is designed to pick up the signs of an ASC as early as possible by asking you (the parents or carers) a few key questions about how the child acts in certain circumstances and then by the health visitor/general practitioner making a few simple requests of the child to elicit certain types of response. (You can get a copy of this checklist from your health visitor or view/download it from various websites.)

Like most developmental disorders, the diagnosis of autism and ASCs is based exclusively on descriptions and observations of past and present behaviour. Although autism, or ASCs, may occur in the context of other, biologically detectable conditions, such as fragile-X and tuberous sclerosis complex (TSC) the specific 'autism' components remain behaviourally defined. There is currently no diagnostic biological test for autism.

This creates an immediate and obvious challenge: which behaviours are characteristic of autism and how many of them must a person 'display' in order to reach the criteria for a diagnosis?

As a so-called 'spectrum' disorder, the individual presentation of autism and an ASC varies widely from one individual to the next. The range of associated strengths and difficulties is such that the very description of autism as a 'disorder' is disputed by many people, who consider their autism as a positive personality trait, whereas others find the condition substantially disabling.

Two sets of diagnostic guidelines are commonly referred to. One is produced by the World Health Organization and incorporated in the International Classification of Diseases (ICD) now in version ten (ICD-10, *The ICD-10 classification of mental and behavioural disorders: clinical descriptions and diagnostic guidelines*, WHO, Geneva). The second is produced by the American Psychiatric Association (APA) and published as the *Diagnostic and Statistical Manual of Mental Disorder* (DSM) now in version four (DSM-IV, *Diagnostic and Statistical Manual of Mental Disorders*, fourth edn (text revision), American Psychiatric Association, 2000). The two sets of guidelines are broadly similar. DSM-IV is used in both the US and the UK while ICD-10 is used in the UK and worldwide.

DSM-IV (American Psychiatric Association)

Pervasive developmental disorder as a diagnostic category appears in DSM-IV in the section named 'Disorders Usually First

Diagnosed in Infancy, Childhood or Adolescence'. The possible diagnoses comprise:

- Autistic disorder (the closest category in DSM-IV to 'classic autism')
- Rett's disorder
- Childhood disintegrative disorder (CDD)
- Asperger's syndrome
- Pervasive developmental disorder – not otherwise specified (PDD-NOS)

For your child to be diagnosed with autism there must be difficulties in all three areas of the autism 'triad of impairments': (a) social interaction; (b) communication; and (c) restricted repetitive (see pages xvii–xviii) and stereotyped patterns of behaviour. Onset must be at or before 36 months of age in at least one of these three areas.

There are additional and very specific requirements to differentiate Rett's disorder and CDD from autistic disorder, and these are relatively rare diagnoses.

For Asperger's syndrome, the requirements include impairment in social interaction and repetitive stereotyped behaviours, but with no speech/language delay and no significant delay in cognitive development, self-help skills or adaptive behaviour.

While many individuals with an Asperger's diagnosis do have substantial communication difficulties, these are not specified in the diagnostic criteria and relate more to pragmatic or social aspects of language. For a diagnosis of Asperger's syndrome the difficulties encountered must also cause clinically significant impairment in social, occupational or other areas of functioning.

A diagnosis of PDD-NOS is used when there is severe and pervasive impairment in the development of reciprocal social interaction, associated with either (a) verbal or non-verbal communication skills, or (b) the presence of stereotyped behaviours, interests and activities that otherwise do not meet the criteria for a specific PDD (for example, autistic disorder). This includes atypical presentations that do not meet criteria for autistic disorder because of late age of onset, atypical symptoms, symptoms that nearly meet the criteria, or all three of these.

Autism spectrum condition

In common with PDD, a diagnosis of an ASC is used to denote a presentation which includes difficulties in social interaction with at least one of (a) communication difficulties; and (b) repetitive stereotyped, restricted patterns of behaviour. Beyond this, and in the absence of additional information, the term is non-specific. In other words, a diagnosis of an ASC does not necessarily mean that the child's presentation is different from 'classic' autism, or in any way atypical. It is crucial, therefore, that at the point of diagnosis the patient (or parent) seeks additional information from the diagnosing clinician about whether or not the child meets the criteria for childhood autism/autistic disorder or not, and if not, what other diagnostic label best describes their presentation.

Sub-types of autism and ASC

Most people are aware that the autism spectrum covers a range of presentations from very mild to very severe. Furthermore, within them there may be unusual characteristics that stand out from the child's other abilities and behaviours. Some very severely affected individuals, for example, have clear areas of extreme giftedness, whereas those who are less severely affected, and who generally function very well, may have some isolated but profound difficulties in areas that many would take for granted.

One important common factor brings all the various ASC presentations together: anyone with an accurate diagnosis of an ASC must have difficulties in social interaction. These difficulties may be accompanied by communication problems and/or by repetitive and restricted patterns of behaviour, but regardless of other behaviours, all adults and children with an ASC, at least according to current diagnostic criteria, have social difficulties. If social difficulties are not present, a diagnosis on the autism spectrum would not be accurate. Typical social difficulties include the inability to make and maintain friendships, poor understanding of social cues, awkward or unusual social approaches and responses, and over-focusing on things of little interest to potential social partners.

Conversely, although when following diagnostic criteria to the letter it is possible to define ASC presentations with social problems alone, social difficulties are almost always accompanied by impairments in communication and repetitive behaviours, or both. Any child or adult who has social problems alone, but who communicates well and who has no indications of repetitive or stereotyped behaviours, is not likely to receive a diagnosis on the autism spectrum.

In reality, therefore, a diagnosis of an ASC means that the person has difficulties with social interaction together with communication problems and/or repetitive, restrictive patterns of behaviour:

Childhood autism/autistic condition is diagnosed when the individual has problems in all three areas, with onset prior to 36 months. Please see the full diagnostic criteria at the end of this chapter.

Atypical autism or PDD-NOS is diagnosed when social problems are present but not all areas of the triad are impaired and/or onset is later than 36 months.

Two diagnoses which are somewhat less well defined are Asperger's syndrome and high-functioning autism:

Asperger's syndrome tends to be diagnosed when there is no significant delay in the development of speech and when general ability/IQ is at or above average levels but when problems in each area of the triad are nonetheless present. Asperger's syndrome is also preferred when the individual demonstrates additional non-autistic problems such as anxiety, motor problems (characteristic of those seen in dyspraxia, for example) and other non-defined psychiatric issues.

High-functioning autism tends to be diagnosed when the individual presents with behaviours more characteristic of classic autism, with difficulties in each area of the triad but with an ability to function well, with at least some cognitive abilities within the normal range and with an absence of the 'non-autistic' problem behaviours seen in Asperger's syndrome.

Why is diagnosis important?

Given the lack of clarity in diagnostic guidelines and the overlap between ASC sub-types, it seems reasonable to ask whether and how a formal diagnosis is useful. A formal diagnosis brings clear advantages, with some potential difficulties and, in general, most practitioners would argue that the former substantially outweigh the latter.

First, a diagnosis provides a means by which a person's difficulties and needs are communicated in a kind of shorthand. If told that a child or adult has an ASC, many people nowadays will understand that the person is likely to have at least some social difficulties, problems with communication and/or a need for a routine and a structured environment. More formally, a diagnosis carries with it the suggestion that additional resources will be needed if the person is to reach their full potential in terms of educational, vocational or occupational achievement.

Although it is not currently guaranteed, a child in the UK who has an ASC diagnosis is also likely to be assessed for a formal statement of special educational needs (a SEN statement) under the Education Act 1996; the more severe the presentation, the more likely this will be. In these circumstances the child is assessed and his or her educational needs will be identified and made explicit. If these are considered significant, they are included in the formal SEN Statement. This brings with it a statutory requirement for the identified needs to be addressed using specific, state-funded provision, together with re-evaluation taking place at least annually.

What to expect from a diagnostic assessment

When a young child or adolescent is diagnosed you will normally find that, as a bare minimum, you will be asked about his or her developmental history and behaviour, but you should also expect the diagnosing clinician to spend time with your child directly, not only in the clinic but also during a routine social setting, such as at school or college. If this isn't possible, reports from the school or college staff should be sought, either by the diagnosing clinician speaking to them directly or by asking them to complete standardised questionnaires.

Where to go for a diagnosis

In the UK, diagnostic evaluations of children or adults are carried out by chartered psychologists (including clinical psychologists and others with relevant expertise), psychiatrists and paediatricians. As a general rule, expect the assessment to extend to beyond the areas required for an ASC diagnosis, so that those working with the individual concerned can plan the appropriate therapeutic and educational strategies. Specialist NHS clinics will often provide a multi-disciplinary team assessment, which may involve cognitive/psychometric specialists, speech and language therapists, occupational and other specialised therapists and educational service providers, who will all have important contributions to make following the diagnostic assessment.

Outside the NHS, diagnostic evaluation is available from the same group of professionals in the private sector but this is likely also to be accompanied by nutritional and biomedical assessments in addition to the more traditional disciplines provided by multi-disciplinary teams within the NHS.

DIAGNOSTIC CRITERIA IN FULL

The following guidelines are published by the American Psychiatric Association (APA) and the World Health Organization (ICD-10) for use when making a diagnosis.

DSM-IV-TR

(The diagnostic criteria for DSM-IV-TR have been reprinted with permission from the *Diagnostic and Statistical Manual of Mental Disorders*, Fourth Edition, Text Revision (Copyright 2000), American Psychiatric Association.)

299.00: Autistic disorder

A. A total of six (or more) items from (1), (2) and (3), with at least two from (1), and one each from (2) and (3):

1. Qualitative impairment in social interaction, as manifested by at least two of the following:

   a. Marked impairment in the use of multiple non-verbal behaviours such as eye-to-eye gaze, facial expression, body postures and gestures to regulate social interaction.

   b. Failure to develop peer relationships appropriate to developmental level.

   c. A lack of spontaneous seeking to share enjoyment, interests or achievements with other people (for example, by a lack of showing, bringing or pointing out objects of interest).

   d. Lack of social or emotional reciprocity.

2. Qualitative impairments in communication as manifested by at least one of the following:

   a. Delay in, or total lack of, the development of spoken language (not accompanied by an attempt to compensate through alternative modes of communication such as gestures or mime).

   b. In individuals with adequate speech, marked impairment in the ability to initiate or sustain a conversation with others.

   c. Stereotyped and repetitive use of language or idiosyncratic language.

   d. Lack of varied, spontaneous make-believe play or social imitative play appropriate to the developmental level.

3. Restricted repetitive and stereotyped patterns of behaviour, interests and activities, as manifested by at least one of the following:

   a. Encompassing preoccupation with one or more stereotyped and restricted patterns of interest that is abnormal either in intensity or focus.

   b. Apparently inflexible adherence to specific, non-functional routines or rituals.

   c. Stereotyped and repetitive motor mannerisms (for example, hand or finger flapping or twisting, or complex whole-body movements).

   d. Persistent preoccupation with parts of objects.

B. Delays or abnormal functioning in at least one of the following areas, with onset prior to age three years: (1) social interaction; (2) language as used in social communication; or (3) symbolic or imaginative play.

C. The disturbance is not better accounted for by Rett's disorder or childhood disintegrative disorder.

299.80: Asperger's disorder

A. Qualitative impairment in social interaction, as manifested by at least two of the following:

1. Marked impairment in the use of multiple non-verbal behaviours such as eye-to-eye gaze, facial expression, body postures, and gestures to regulate social interaction.

2. Failure to develop peer relationships appropriate to developmental level.

3. A lack of spontaneous seeking to share enjoyment, interests, or achievements with other people (for example, by a lack of showing, bringing or pointing out objects of interest to other people).

B. Restricted repetitive and stereotyped patterns of behaviour, interests, and activities, as manifested by at least one of the following:

1. Encompassing preoccupation with one or more stereotyped and restricted patterns of interest that is abnormal either in intensity or focus.

2. Apparently inflexible adherence to specific, non-functional routines or rituals.

3. Stereotyped and repetitive motor mannerisms (for example, hand or finger flapping or twisting, or complex whole-body movements).

4. Persistent preoccupation with parts of objects.

C. The disturbance causes clinically significant impairment in social, occupational or other important areas of functioning.

D. There is no clinically significant general delay in language (for example, single words used by age two years, communicative phrases used by age three years).

E. There is no clinically significant delay in cognitive development or in the development of age-appropriate self-help skills, adaptive behaviour (other than in social interaction) and curiosity about the environment in childhood.

F. Criteria are not met for another specific pervasive developmental disorder or schizophrenia.

299.00: Pervasive developmental disorder not otherwise specified (including atypical autism)

This category should be used when there is a severe and pervasive impairment in the development of reciprocal social interaction associated with impairment in either verbal or nonverbal communication skills or with the presence of stereotyped behaviour, interest, and activities, but the criteria are not met for a specific pervasive developmental disorder, schizophrenia, schizotypal personality disorder, or avoidant personality disorder; for example, this category includes atypical autism – presentations that do not meet the criteria for autistic disorder because of late age at onset, atypical symptomatology or sub-threshold symptomatology, or all of these.

ICD-10
(The diagnostic criteria for ICD-10 have been reprinted with permission from the World Health Organization.)

F84: Pervasive developmental disorders
A group of disorders characterised by qualitative abnormalities in reciprocal social interactions and in patterns of communication, and by a restricted, stereotyped, repetitive repertoire of interests and activities. These qualitative abnormalities are a pervasive feature of the individual's functioning in all situations.

Use additional code, if desired, to identify any associated medical condition and mental retardation.

F84.0: Childhood autism
A type of pervasive developmental disorder defined by:

a. The presence of abnormal or impaired development manifested before the age of three years.

b. The characteristic type of abnormal functioning in all the three areas of psychopathology: reciprocal social interaction, communication and restricted, stereotyped, repetitive behaviour.

In addition, a range of other non-specific problems are common, such as phobias, sleeping and eating disturbances, temper tantrums, and (self-directed) aggression.

Autistic disorder
Infantile:

- Autism

- Psychosis

Kanner's syndrome

Excludes: autistic psychopathy (F84.5) (Asperger's Syndrome)

F84.1: Atypical autism
A type of pervasive developmental disorder that differs from childhood autism either in age of onset or in failing to fulfil all three sets of diagnostic criteria. This sub-category should be used when there is abnormal and impaired development that is present only after age three years, and a lack of sufficient demonstrable abnormalities in one or two of the three areas of psychopathology required for the diagnosis of autism (namely, reciprocal social interactions, communication and restricted, stereotyped, repetitive behaviour) in spite of characteristic abnormalities in the other area(s). Atypical autism arises most often in profoundly retarded individuals and in individuals with a severe specific developmental disorder of receptive language.

Atypical childhood psychosis. Mental retardation with autistic features.

Use additional code (F70–F79), if desired, to identify mental retardation.

F84.2: Rett's syndrome

A condition, so far found only in girls, in which apparently normal early development is followed by partial or complete loss of speech and of skills in locomotion and use of hands, together with deceleration in head growth, usually with an onset between 7 and 24 months of age. Loss of purposive hand movements, hand-wringing stereotypes, and hyperventilation are characteristic. Social and play development are arrested but social interest tends to be maintained. Trunk ataxia (see note 1) and apraxia (see note 2) start to develop by age four years and choreoathetoid (see note 3) movements frequently follow. Severe mental retardation almost invariably results.

F84.3: Other childhood disintegrative disorder

A type of pervasive developmental disorder that is defined by a period of entirely normal development before the onset of the disorder, followed by a definite loss of previously acquired skills in several areas of development over the course of a few months. Typically, this is accompanied by a general loss of interest in the environment, by stereotyped, repetitive motor mannerisms, and by autistic-like abnormalities in social interaction and communication. In some cases the disorder can be shown to be due to some associated encephalopathy but the diagnosis should be made on the behavioural features.

Dementia infantilis

Disintegrative psychosis

Heller's syndrome

Symbiotic psychosis

Excludes Rett's syndrome (F84.2)

F84.4: Overactive disorder associated with mental retardation and stereotyped movements

An ill-defined disorder of uncertain nosological (see note 4) validity. The category is designed to include a group of children with severe mental retardation (IQ below 35) who show major problems in hyperactivity and in attention, as well as stereotyped behaviours. They tend not to benefit from stimulant drugs (unlike those with an IQ in the normal range) and may exhibit a severe dysphoric (see note 5) reaction (sometimes with psychomotor retardation) when given stimulants. In adolescence, the overactivity tends to be replaced by underactivity (a pattern that is not usual in hyperkinetic children with normal intelligence). This syndrome is also often associated with a variety of developmental delays, either specific or global. The extent to which the behavioural pattern is a function of low IQ or of organic brain damage is not known.

F84.5: Asperger's syndrome

A disorder of uncertain nosological-4 validity, characterised by the same type of qualitative abnormalities of reciprocal social interaction that typify autism, together with a restricted, stereotyped, repetitive repertoire of interests and activities. It differs from autism primarily in the fact that there is no general delay or retardation in language or in cognitive development. This disorder is often associated with marked clumsiness. There is a strong tendency for the abnormalities to persist into adolescence and adult life. Psychotic episodes occasionally occur in early adult life.

Autistic psychopathy

Schizoid disorder of childhood

F84.8: Other pervasive developmental disorders

F84.9: Pervasive developmental disorder, unspecified

See notes overleaf

Notes

1. Ataxia is a neurological condition involving the loss of control of coordination and body movements.

2. Apraxia is a neurological condition involving an inability to perform deliberate physical movements.

3. Choreoathetoid movements are involuntary and purposeless movements of the limbs, face and body that are both jerky (choreic) and writhing (athetoid).

4. Nosology is the branch of medical science concerned with the classification of disease.

5. Dysphoria is a state of anxiety, depression, unhappiness or general malaise, the opposite of euphoria.

So, with Billy's diagnosis of autism in place, it was time to look at why our boy was so sick. At no point in any literature (limited as it then was) did it say that bowel problems like those Billy was presenting were part of the condition of autism. Jon started to look at why our little boy was so desperately sick, and what he discovered is described in the next chapter.

CHAPTER 3

The Gut–Brain Connection

This is one of the most important chapters in this book, as there is growing evidence that a positive link exists between the gut, which is often referred to as the second brain, and the way in which the brain functions. Surrounding the gut is the enteric nervous system, the second largest mass of nerve cells in the human body after the brain. The gut has a very close relationship with the brain, sharing many receptors and neurotransmitters. The vagus nerve also connects the two organs and it is understood that toxins may pass from the gut to the brain and alter the way in which it functions. The health and function of the gut is vital to the functioning of the brain. Identifying the hidden problems in the gut and treating them accordingly will lead to better physical and mental health. Over 92 per cent of the individuals diagnosed with an ASC that I see in my clinic have gut-related disturbances, and this was no different for my son. Identifying the causes of his gut dysfunction and addressing each individually has led Billy to achieve so much more. Because Billy's gut problems have been corrected, his autism, including his social problems and behaviours, have all improved and, most importantly, he is now living without any gut-related problems.

Billy's gut history

The day after Billy's MMR vaccination at 13 months, he developed chronic diarrhoea, which lasted for 18 months. This significant and dramatic change in his gut function marked the beginning of his deterioration into autism.

During that 18-month period, his weight plummeted, dropping from the 97th percentile to the seventh, he lost condition, his stomach was bloated, he developed eczema and his hair started to fall out (alopecia). He lost all his baby speech, slipped away from us and became isolated in his own world.

As we've explained, Billy had suffered recurrent chest and ear infections for six months up to his first birthday, all treated with antibiotics, but seemingly to no avail. Knowing what we know now, it seems likely that an allergy or intolerance to dairy may have contributed significantly to his excessive mucus production, and it's clear that the relentless antibiotic assault on his developing immune system and gut flora left him severely immunosuppressed, increasingly unable to fight off infection and actually more vulnerable to opportunistic pathogens. This led to many gut-related problems, and this is significant to what happened to his brain and the way it functioned.

Dr Natasha Campbell-McBride, in her 2003 book *Gut and Psychology Syndrome: Natural Treatment for Dyspraxia, Autism, ADD, Dyslexia, ADHD, Depression, Schizophrenia*, sums up the issue as follows: 'A baby is born with an immature immune system. Establishment of healthy balanced gut flora in the first few days of life plays a crucial role in appropriate maturation of the immune system. If the baby does not acquire appropriate gut flora then the baby is left immune compromised.' This compromised immune system then allows infection to occur. Antibiotics are then commonly prescribed and the child's health further deteriorates making him or her even more susceptible to attack from bad bacteria and other pathogens.

Billy's gut issues were dismissed by his doctors: 'he's got toddler diarrhoea' said one, 'he eats too many apples' said another and, believe this, 'of course he has diarrhoea – he has autism' said another. I still find it hard to believe that a diagnosis of autism can be so readily associated with bowel problems but dismissed in such a blasé manner and that this association seems to preclude the further investigation that would be afforded to any other child who had the same chronic symptoms.

One treatment we tried for Billy was the introduction of secretin given intravenously (secretin is a hormone derived from the pancreas that controls the secretions in the small intestine as well as supporting its pH balance). The treatment led to Billy's first normal stool in 18 months and, with that, greater focus and concentration, better eye contact, improved socialisation and an ability to try a greater range of foods. (For full details about secretin and our experiences with it see pages 72–4.) This confirmed our suspicions that some form of gut dysfunction was pertinent to his autism, or at least to the severity of the symptoms we've come to associate with the condition.

What happens when gut function is compromised?

If gut function is impaired, there is a breakdown in digestion and the absorption of proteins, fats, carbohydrates, vitamins and minerals. Through conducting a comprehensive digestive stool analysis (CDSA) we found that Billy had low levels of vital acid secretions in his stomach. He had limited nutrient absorption and deficiencies in vitamins A, B_1, B_3, B_6, B_{12}, C, chromium, magnesium, manganese, selenium and zinc. He also had inflammation and a number of additional problems associated with candidiasis, parasitic infection and poor digestion of proteins. The functions of the deficient vitamins and minerals (as well as all the others) are many and varied, but you'll find them all in the vitamin and mineral charts in the Appendix.

The CDSA test also found two pathogenic parasites (*Blasto-cystis hominis* and *Dientamoeba fragilis*) present in Billy's gut. These amoebic parasites are associated with multiple gut symptoms including abdominal pain, inflammation, flatulence, diarrhoea, vomiting and weight loss. Many authorities believe that the presence of amoebic parasites and the symptoms they cause are often misdiagnosed as irritable bowel syndrome (IBS). Unfortunately, the dramatic implications of these two remark-ably common parasites are still a matter of debate within the medical fraternity, and they are unlikely to be picked up or acknowledged in routine testing.

Identifying gut symptoms

I do hope you will learn a lot from this chapter about the gut and the problems that many of our children with an ASC commonly experience. Many issues associated with the gut also cause pain; they hurt, and you must always be aware of this, especially in those children whose language is limited so that they cannot tell you where it hurts, and who may react to the pain in any number of different ways.

Signs of pain

You need to become aware of the manifestations of a multi-tude of gut-related problems that signify pain, discomfort and illness: strange postures, bloated tummies, poor 'ability to thrive', poor muscle tone, weird behaviours like lying across the edge of a table or the arm of a chair, crying for no apparent reason, red ear lobes, food fads and intense dislikes, sensitivities to texture, bad breath, red itchy bottom, worms, stool (poo) problems like constipation and diarrhoea, partic-ularly smelly stools, undigested foods in the stool, sometimes light and sometimes dark stools, grains in the stool and rectal bleeding (the list goes on). These are just some of the observable effects that represent possible gut-related issues that need addressing.

Autism and the gut

It is well known that gut-related disturbances are very common in individuals with autism, and therefore if the gut is not functioning optimally, then perhaps neither will the brain. We know that the majority of toxins we are exposed to are absorbed by the gut and taken into our blood system and circulated around the body. We know that everything that is absorbed across the gut membrane is taken to the liver for detoxification. We know that many individuals with an ASC have liver stress and a poor ability to get rid of toxins due to low levels of glutathione; also, because of nutrient deficiencies, there is a breakdown in some of the reactions, and some of the compounds that enable our bodies to eliminate toxins are reduced. For Billy, the identification and treatment of gut-related problems was the start of his healing.

These issues are not to be taken for granted or rationalised as 'part of the condition'; they are symptoms of an underlying serious health condition that may be exacerbating the symptoms of your child's autism, and could even have caused or triggered it – and many of them are treatable. You *can* make it better.

Dr Brian Jepson, physician and parent of a child with autism, writes in *Changing the Course of Autism: A Scientific Approach to Treating your Autistic Child* that 'autism is an environmental illness with a genetic component'. He goes on to say that autism is treatable, but is a very complicated illness: 'Our children are trapped in there and we have to fight to get them back out.'

The gut is extremely susceptible to damage from a range of outside influences: from antibiotic treatments, from the effects of a poor diet, non-steroidal drugs such as ibuprofen, from stress and from anything that might cause an imbalance in the gut flora.

In order to understand the true implications of these variables, I'm going to take you through the key points of digestion and basic nutrition so that what I will go on to say about the implications of gastrointestinal disorders and nutrition in people with autism will make more sense.

In this book I will give you advice and practical suggestions about how to address various digestive issues through the diet, so you need to have a basic understanding of the digestive process.

The digestive system

Digestion is the breakdown of foods eaten and the absorption of the nutrients contained therein to be available for all bodily processes and chemical reactions:

1. The digestive process starts in the mouth. Food is moved around in the mouth by the tongue, broken up by chewing, and mixed with saliva. Saliva contains two enzymes: amylase, which starts to break starch down into sugar, and lysozyme, which kills bacteria. The chewed food then is swallowed via the gullet (oesophagus) and taken into the stomach.

2. Once food enters the stomach, the muscles in the stomach wall contract and relax to 'churn' the food and mix it with gastric juices: a mixture of mucus, stomach acid (hydrochloric acid), gastric juice and digestive enzymes (mainly pepsin, trypsin and lipase).

3. The acid creates the optimum environment for the enzymes to work, helps digest the food and kills off most of the remaining harmful bacteria. Pepsin breaks proteins down into peptides, lipase breaks certain fats down, and mucus lubricates and helps to protect the stomach lining from the acid.

4. After a couple of hours in the stomach, a valve opens, allowing small amounts of partially digested food into the duodenum – the first part of the small intestine. The acid content of this food material (the chyme) stimulates the pancreas to release digestive enzymes and bicarbonate ions to neutralise the acidity, preventing 'burning' of the small intestine and to help set up the correct pH environment for the beneficial bacteria to colonise and live.

5. The small intestine is responsible for completing the digestion of foods by secreting enzymes and also by the work done by the beneficial bacteria.

6. Bile, with waste toxins from the body extracted from the blood system by the liver, helps to emulsify fats (breaking them down into microscopic droplets that mix more readily with water), enabling them to be absorbed into the lymphatic and blood systems.

7. The waste matter that cannot be digested or absorbed then passes into the large intestine, which is where most of the water is absorbed to keep us hydrated.

8. Once the chyme has reached the large intestine, the digestion process is practically complete and most of the nutrients have been absorbed. Almost all that is left are the indigestible parts of food: mostly dietary fibre from fruit and vegetables.

9. The main function of the colon (the large intestine) is to absorb any remaining water (and some minerals and salts) from the indigestible waste. This waste is mixed with more mucus and acted on by bacteria from the colonies that live in the large intestine (the gut flora) to extract any remaining nutrients, while feeding themselves and fermenting soluble fibre and any remaining food residue (creating methane gas as a

bi-product). The waste is converted to solid waste (faeces) and moves on to the rectum ready for excretion.

10. The whole process of digestion can take 24 hours or more, depending on the type of food you've eaten.

Gut flora – why is it so important?

As I explained earlier, the human digestive tract (the gut) contains literally trillions of bacteria. These are known collectively as the gut flora. These complex colonies of microorganisms serve a vital purpose in the body's immune system: keeping us healthy by suppressing or warding off bacterial, fungal, parasitic and viral pathogens (germs) and toxins, preventing them from spreading or penetrating through the gut wall to cause infection or disease. They also play a part in the digestion and absorption of food and nutrients, fermenting soluble fibre into short-chain fatty acids and synthesising B vitamins, and so on.

Human health, digestion, immune function and metabolic balance depend to such an extent upon maintaining colonies of good bacteria that some people consider the gut flora to constitute an organ in its own right.

Secretory IgA

The beneficial bacteria described above stimulate the production of secretory immunoglobulin A (sec IgA), which is the immune system's main defensive antibody against invading pathogens. Approximately 70–80 per cent of our total immune 'army' resides in the gut.

Sec IgA is also an important component of the paste that coats the beneficial bacteria, preventing them from coming into direct contact with the cell walls and therefore avoiding an immune response. A lack of sec IgA can therefore cause further immune responses, leading to inflammation and cellular damage.

Dysbiosis

An imbalance in the gut flora leading to the overgrowth of harmful bacteria and yeast in the gut is known as dysbiosis. Many people believe that dysbiosis lies at the root of many serious health complaints such as IBS, chronic fatigue, eczema, multiple sclerosis and rheumatoid arthritis, and this is common among individuals with an ASC.

The body's supply of good bacteria can be adversely affected by a number of factors: some diseases, the effects of stress, poor diet and, particularly, the use of antibiotics can deplete gut flora colonies, wiping out large numbers of good bacteria and thereby reducing the gut's defences against illness and infection caused by bad bacteria, parasites, viruses and yeasts.

The use of antibiotics can therefore impair the gut flora's ability to self-regulate by suppressing bad bacteria and may lead to a range of secondary infections, two of the most common being the diarrhoea and colitis (inflammation of the colon) caused by the bacterium *Clostridium difficile* and yeast infections (candidiasis) caused by *Candida albicans*, both of which are normally suppressed by the natural dominance of good bacteria in the gut.

There are many factors that can upset the delicate balance of the gut flora and gastrointestinal (GI) tract:

- Immune system dysfunction with low sec IgA production
- Frequent use of antibiotics
- Changes in gut pH
- Food allergies
- Non-steroidal anti-inflammatory drugs, such as ibuprofen
- Parasitic infection
- Viral infection
- Excessive stress
- Excessive toxins including heavy metals
- Poor diet: rich in refined carbohydrates, saturated fats and sugar

- Insufficient fibre within the diet
- Overgrowth of yeast, particularly *Candida* species
- The presence of a biofilm (explained later)

If there's one thing that's clear, it's that all the various factors of diet, metabolism and immune function are inter-related and interdependent. It should be glaringly obvious by now that the delicate balance of all the body systems can have dramatic implications on overall health and well-being. There is plenty of evidence to suggest that many of the factors involving the relationship between gut health and brain function are particularly relevant to people with an ASC.

As previously mentioned, I have seen more than 500 children in my autism clinic and have found that 92 per cent have had three or more of the gastrointestinal problems listed below, indicating that the gut plays a major role in autism:

- Diarrhoea
- Constipation
- Foul-smelling stools
- Particularly light or dark stools
- Mucus present in the stool
- Increased intestinal permeability, or leaky gut
- Undigested food in the stool
- Parasites
- Dysbiosis and elevated proprionic acid level
- Biofilm presence

In addition to these, let me highlight a few other associated disturbances and pertinent issues that I have identified in the children I am supporting through the Autism Clinic:

- Bloatedness/abdominal distension/increased flatus (wind).
- Inadequate enzyme function, especially enzymes that break down proteins into amino acids (called proteases).

- The presence of parasites, pathogenic bacteria such as streptococcal, staphylococcal and clostridial species, yeasts (especially *Candida*) and viruses, often arising from gut-flora imbalance: dysbiosis.
- Sec IgA disturbances and inflammation.
- Disturbed pH levels – either too alkaline or too acidic.
- Inadequate hydrochloric acid production in the stomach (vital for a number of digestive and metabolic processes).
- Poor digestion and absorption of nutrients – low levels of amino acids, essential fatty acids, minerals, vitamins and trace elements.
- High levels of proprionic acid released by bad bacteria (proprionic acid has been found to cause autistic behaviour in rats).
- Elevated levels of arabinose – an indicator of candidiasis.

Dr Karoly S. Horvath, director of the Pediatric Gastrointestinal and Nutrition Laboratory at the University of Maryland, Baltimore, USA wrote: 'Recent clinical studies have revealed a high prevalence of gastrointestinal symptoms, inflammation and dysfunction in children with autism. Mild to moderate degrees of inflammation were found in the upper and lower intestinal tract.' ('Autistic disorder and gastrointestinal disease', *Paediatrics*, vol. 14, (2002): 583–7.)

Stools

Many, if not most, of these gut issues, either individually or collectively, will affect the way that the stool (faeces) is formed in the bowel. Unpleasant though it may be, you can read quite a lot from the consistency of your child's poo.

The Bristol Stool Chart is widely used as a simple tool for categorising types of stool. It presents seven stool types, ranging in form and consistency from constipation to diarrhoea:

Type 1 Separate, hard lumps, like nuts (hard to pass).

Type 2 Sausage-shaped but lumpy (and hard).

Type 3 Like a sausage, but with cracks on its surface.

Type 4 Like a sausage or snake, smooth and soft.

Type 5 Soft blobs with clear-cut edges (passed easily).

Type 6 Fluffy pieces with ragged edges, a mushy stool.

Type 7 Watery, no solid pieces; entirely liquid.

Ideally, every stool passed should conform to types 3 or 4. Anything above that (that is, 1 and 2) indicates constipation; and anything below (5, 6 and 7) indicates varying degrees of diarrhoea. You don't have to go into it any further than this, but if your child's stool is regularly 1–2 or 5–7, then something is going wrong and this will help in the investigation of any underlying causes.

I have had one child in my clinic who passed nothing but a type 1 stool every eight days and was frightened of going. This doesn't surprise me, as a type 1 stool would be painful to pass. The recurrence of such issues, particularly at an early age, can set up all sorts of psychological barriers to 'normal' toileting, let alone the obvious physical ones, and will tend to indicate gut disorders that might be causing all kinds of other issues, such as pain and discomfort.

As a general rule, the form of the stool is directly related to how long it has spent in the colon (large intestine/bowel) and how much water has been absorbed from the faecal mass. A harder stool means it is drier, because it has been in the gut for longer; it may also mean that there is a large amount of insoluble fibre or insufficient fluids have been drunk, causing dehydration, or it may be that peristalsis is weak. A softer, wetter stool indicates poor water absorption and irritation causing the gut to eliminate the cause of the irritation – whether they be toxins or bacteria, and so on.

Many of the persistent and familiar pathogens that we've discussed can result in diarrhoea or constipation, so it would be crazy not to consider their effects if your child consistently passes the wrong kind of stool. The functioning of the gut is inextricably linked with the food you eat, the stress you're under, the efficiency (or otherwise) of your immune system and, of course, the balance of gut flora, so anything that seems out of the ordinary (that is, not a type 3 or 4) means that something is awry and should be investigated.

Billy's multiple courses of antibiotics from 6 to 12 months certainly would not have helped the status of his gut flora. Antibiotics reduced the beneficial bacteria in his gut and set up dysbiosis and further suppressed his immune system. By completing an IgM antibody test, Billy was found to have measles in his gut; I have to ask myself, therefore, was this a result of an immune system that was already dysfunctional before the MMR was given, enabling measles to become active in his body? This would seem to emphasise the risks of susceptibility in some babies posed by a genetic predisposition. This will affect their ability to deal with toxins, and if their immune system is compromised, their ability to deal with pathogens, such as bacteria and viruses, will be reduced and they may also be more sensitive to allergens.

Allergic conditions

Many parents with a child diagnosed with autism who have completed my detailed questionnaire themselves have a history of atopic health issues, such as asthma and hay fever, autoimmune disease and food intolerance. ('Atopic' refers to allergic conditions that present symptoms in parts of the body not in direct contact with the allergen that caused them.) This disrupts the balance of specific white blood cells, called Th1 and Th2 helper cells, making the body less protected against infectious agents such as bacteria and viruses. The child will also be more susceptible to certain immune responses such as food intolerances or allergies and will be compromised in dealing with pathogenic exposure to viruses, bacteria, parasites and fungal species.

Intestinal permeability or leaky gut (explained on page 57) can result from dysbiosis, whereby pathogenic bacterial species,

Candida, parasites and viruses are running wild in a poorly protected gut due to the inefficient immune response against them. This then leads to increased localised inflammation and gut-tissue damage, plus resulting toxicity, increased allergen exposure and an increase in inflammation elsewhere in the body due to the pathogens and food peptides being able to leak through the normally impermeable gut wall. Some of the more commonly found species that produce toxins that can affect the brain are listed below:

Candida (yeast species)

In addition to the well-known implications of *Candida* in the general population (tummy bugs, oral and vaginal thrush, and so on), *Candida* species are known to be particularly problematical in individuals with autism. They produce a whole range of mycotoxins (fungal poisons) as waste products. The resulting symptoms vary widely, but can include fatigue, mood swings, depression, the inability to concentrate, headaches, loss of energy, food cravings, mould sensitivity, multiple food and chemical intolerances and nervous-system problems.

Clostridium difficile

The bacterium *Clostridium difficile* is prevalent in people with an ASC and is a major bacterial culprit in gut disturbances, particularly diarrhoea and colitis, ranging from mild disturbance to very severe illness. The Clostridia family include the bacteria that cause tetanus (see below), botulism and gangrene.

Clostridium tetani

Back in 1998, Ellen Bolte, parent, researcher and microbiologist, outlined the possibility of a serious tetanus infection of the gut being an underlying cause of autism in some individuals.

Clostridium tetani is a bacillus known to produce a potent neurotoxin: proprionic acid. The normal site of binding for the toxin is the spinal cord; however, the vagus nerve (a lengthy nerve 'strand' that carries information to and fro between the brain and various body organs) is capable of transporting tetanus neuro-toxin, thus providing a route from the intestinal tract to the central nervous system and thus bypassing the spinal cord. Once in the brain it may disrupt the release of neurotransmitters. This may explain the characteristics of some autistic symptoms.

A study conducted in 2000 with 11 children who had autism found that treating Clostridia overgrowth with selective microbial agents (oral vancomycin and metronidazole) led to short-term improvements in their autistic symptoms, indicating a link between Clostridia and autism that is clearly worthy of further dedicated research.

Proprionic acid

Sometimes called propionic or propanoic acid, proprionic acid is a short-chain fatty acid that is a by-product of the fermentation of foodstuffs by some bacteria.

Dr Derrick MacFabe, director of The Autism Research Group at the University of Western Ontario, completed studies on rats by injecting them with proprionic acid, observing that they developed autistic-like behaviours: 'They immediately engaged in bouts of repetitive behaviour, hyperactivity and impaired social behaviours which had close similarity to what parents are seeing with autism.' The rats' brains were later examined and found to contain inflammatory processes similar to those in the brains of children who have autism.

This could be yet another part of the autism puzzle evolving. I have conducted many lab tests on the children I am looking after, and elevated proprionic acid is apparent in over 95 per cent of all cases (found using the Optimal Nutrition Evaluation test).

Again, the presence of proprionic acid is a result of the over-growth of harmful bacterial species that have been allowed to colonise due to a deficient immune system and depleted gut flora. The question of how the overgrowth starts is often relatively simple.

Many parents of children with autism explain how multiple courses of antibiotics have often been prescribed to their children. This is frequently for illnesses early in life such as respiratory tract infections and ear infections; however, after multiple rounds of antibiotics (presumably because of secondary infections or because, for whatever reason, the illness didn't clear up) the normal protective bacteria simply do not exist in sufficient numbers in the gut. This provides a perfect set of conditions for the harmful bacteria to thrive and also for antibiotic-resistant bacteria, parasites, yeasts and viruses and the possibility of a biofilm.

Biofilm

A biofilm is a thin mucous membrane that builds up on the inside of the gut wall.

'Irritants' on the gut surface, such as pathogens – bad bacteria, viruses, parasites and fungal species – plus food allergens, produce an immune response causing inflammation of the gut. The gut membrane produces mucus to 'dampen down' the inflammation and to get rid of the dead cells and debris. Inflammation in these damaged areas also increases the release of a substance called fibrin that is used as a cement to help give some form and solidity to the mucus. Fibrin also uses metals, such as iron, and minerals, such as calcium and magnesium, to help support its structure, rather like steel girders, and it can form a matrix (a structure) capable of hiding pathogens away from the immune system and from being killed by antibiotics. It also reduces the absorption and the availability of nutrients.

Middle-ear infections and glue ear (otitis media and chronic otitis media), which are very common in children diagnosed with an ASC, are being increasingly linked to biofilm presence, which may explain why such infections tend to be resistant to antibiotic treatment.

The bacterial biofilm is alive and continues to leach toxins into the bloodstream while remaining protected from the immune system. If you carry out a stool analysis, these bugs may not even show up. I have completed many stool analyses on the children I see at the clinic and, after some gut-supportive therapy, 'new' bacterial species will appear in the stool specimen results. This is the result of the degradation of the biofilm and the release of these previously hidden bacteria. It is therefore extremely important that this problem is professionally treated to reduce the pathogens present in the gut and to reduce inflammation, as well as enhancing the absorption of nutrients, many of which are deficient in individuals with an ASC.

What is leaky gut syndrome?

Increased intestinal permeability, or leaky gut syndrome, is present in many people with autism and this in particular may place them at an increased risk of food allergy, infection and increased toxicity.

One of the most widely espoused theories about the biomedical aspects of autism and an ASC is that many people with autism have suffered damage to the lining of the intestines, enabling undigested or partially digested proteins (such as gluten and casein) and toxins to enter the bloodstream. This is often referred to as 'leaky gut syndrome', and can be caused by many factors such as an imbalance of gut bacteria, parasites, fungi and viruses creating inflammation, or by the use of non-steroidal anti-inflammatory drugs such as ibuprofen, or by food allergens and poor sulphation. (Sulphation is a series of chemical reactions that strengthen the gut membrane and support the production of our most important antioxidant, glutathione.) This has been identified by Dr Rosemary Waring, a human toxicologist at the University of Birmingham, who found that most people with an ASC were low in sulphate.

Under normal circumstances, the gut wall has a number of effective defences. The first line of defence is the 'army' of helpful bacteria that live on every surface, providing a physical barrier and keeping the bad guys at bay. Then there is the integrity of the gut wall itself: epithelial cells are densely packed, with very tight 'junctions' between them that only allow small molecules to get through.

What are the symptoms associated with leaky gut?

The leakage of partially digested proteins as well as harmful bacteria and toxins into the bloodstream may cause the immune system to treat these molecules as foreign bodies and therefore 'learn' to attack them, leading to the development of food allergies, inflammatory responses and the resultant production of free radicals, which are highly reactive, unstable molecules that cause cellular damage and are implicated in a range of serious health conditions.

One of the most significant consequences of leaky gut is hepatic stress: stress on the liver and its vital detoxification functions. The liver is responsible for filtering out all the toxins, pathogens and undigested food particles that make it through the gut wall and into the bloodstream. The more toxins, and so on, it has to deal with, the more stress will be put on all its functions, including depleting its reserves of sulphur-containing amino acids, such as cysteine and methionine, which are in turn vital to the production of the super-antioxidant, glutathione.

Probably the most familiar aspect of leaky gut syndrome is its association with gluten and casein allergy.

The peptides derived from the proteins in wheat and milk (gluteomorphin/gliadorphin and casomorphin) would, under normal circumstances, be too large to be absorbed through the gut wall into the bloodstream, but are allowed to pass through under the conditions defined by leaky gut syndrome. These peptides act as opioids, where they replicate the effects of opiate drugs and can cause significant problems with speech, communication, behaviour and social skills as well as various other effects similar to those of opiate drugs, including addiction. This may cause some people with an ASC to crave foods that are high in gluten and casein. Some studies have also found that people with an ASC are low in the enzymes (DPP1V) required to digest gluten and casein.

Although there is strong anecdotal evidence for the efficacy of a gluten-free and casein-free (GFCF) diet for some people with an ASC, one recent study has found that people with an ASC do not show abnormally high levels of opioid peptides in their bloodstreams. Given the extraordinary results that some people get after following a GFCF diet, this is puzzling, and may imply that only a particular subset of children with autism, who were not identified in the study, are at risk from this phenomenon, or that some other immunological system is at work here. More research is definitely needed.

Gut problems lead to nutrient deficiencies

Dysbiosis, inflammation, a biofilm and leaky gut can have a dramatic effect on the way that nutrients are absorbed into the bloodstream from the food we eat: damage to the intestinal villi (finger-like projections in the lining to the small intestine) reduces the absorption surface; a leaky gut allows the passage of undigested proteins into the blood system promoting food allergies; a deficiency in beneficial bacteria reduces the digestion of food; and poor sulphation slows the healing process of the gut. The end result is that the body is starved of the nutrients and molecular building blocks it needs so that it can perform a vast array of vital functions. The efficient way in which the food we eat is broken down into individual nutrients and then absorbed by the body is absolutely vital to overall health.

Inflammation, leaky gut, dysbiosis (page 49) and biofilms are all issues commonly associated with individuals with autism. Without the gut functioning optimally, health issues will arise, so these conditions must be treated for health to be restored.

Testing for inflammation and its treatment

Inflammation is caused by two problematical groups: allergens and pathogens (bad guys such as parasites, bacteria, viruses and fungi). In order to reduce inflammation these need to be identified. Food allergens can be isolated via blood screens such as the Food Antigen Cellular Test (available from Genova Diagnostics, although you would need to be referred for this by a medical or nutritional practitioner). There is a simpler and cheaper alternative: the food pulse test.

Food pulse test

1. Take the resting pulse before eating.
2. Take the pulse by placing two or three fingers of one hand about 2.5cm (1in) below the thumb on the wrist. Count the beats for a *full* minute (please note that for this test it is not adequate to time 30 seconds and then to multiply by two).
3. After taking the pulse, place a piece of the test food in the mouth.
4. Chew and hold the food in the mouth for two minutes and then take the pulse again for one minute. If the pulse goes up four beats, the body is sensitive to the food and should only be eaten occasionally. If it goes up eight beats or more, this increase would suggest an allergic reaction.

Treatment for inflammation

The foods that have caused your pulse to increase may also have produced an allergic reaction causing or contributing to inflammation and must be excluded from the diet.

The diet should be changed to one that is as hypo-allergenic (unlikely to cause an allergic reaction) as possible. Diets that are hypo-allergenic are likely to exclude dairy, gluten, nuts, eggs, corn and soy, so are likely to involve a huge disruption to your family routines and your child's favourite foods, so it's worth putting in the time and effort to pin down the actual allergies, intolerances and sensitivities before embarking on such a venture.

The most familiar exclusion diet for people with an ASC is the GFCF diet, but there are also others that may be more suitable, including the specific carbohydrate diet, the body ecology diet, low oxalate diet, low salicylate diet and anti-*Candida* diet. These and others are discussed in Chapter 10.

In my opinion, it is important to offer a diet that is specific to the individual, as not one of the diets listed above will be absolutely correct for every individual with an ASC. The diet should also be used to provide the necessary nutrient and fibre support for the gut to function optimally.

You may need to support the gut flora, the health of the gut membrane, the liver and its abilities to detoxify (see Chapter 5), and you may also need to heal a leaky gut or eradicate a biofilm as and when necessary, following specific identification of the problem.

Testing for leaky gut and its treatment

One of the first things to do is to complete a number of diagnostic tests to ascertain how the gut is functioning, and these are explained in Chapter 4. It is imperative that before treating any problem a thorough investigation is carried out to ascertain exactly what the problem is and the causes behind it. Before healing the leaky gut it is important to test to see if it is present. The most straightforward way to do this is to use the lactulose/mannitol test, which is supplied by many individual laboratories. (You will need to consult a medical or nutritional practitioner to help coordinate this and to provide a detailed interpretation of the results.) The test involves drinking a solution containing two different sugars, lactulose and mannitol. A healthy gut allows the smaller mannitol molecules (a monosaccharide) to be absorbed through the gut wall and into the urine via the kidneys but not the larger lactulose molecules (a disaccharide), which would only be partially absorbed, if at all. If, on testing the urine, it was found to contain high levels of both sugars this would indicate that the gut is leaky.

Treatment for leaky gut

Once you have established through testing what is going on in your child's gut, there are a variety of things you can do to help the healing process. The main aspects to focus on are as follows:

Immune modulation

As previously mentioned, individuals with an ASC have a distorted immune system favouring a dominant Th2 helper cell response (see page 53) so they are great at attacking the allergen but poor at defending themselves against the bad guys, such as bacteria or viruses, due to low levels of the other Th1 helper cell group. They may also have deficiencies in sec IgA (which protects all mucosal barriers such as the gut and lungs) and therefore that will need boosting. If bad guys are living in the gut, it is the compromised immune system or the presence of a biofilm (see page 56) that is allowing them to colonise. Treatments such as antibiotics, antivirals and antifungals have been used with some success in helping the individual manage these overgrowths, but many will return once the treatment is stopped. Enhancing the Th1 response and enhancing the natural production of sec IgA is vital for the immune system to protect the gut.

I always recommend finding a general practitioner and qualified nutritional practitioner who are well versed in treating individuals with autism. They may well prescribe products such as Mycocyclin and PhytoCort by Allergy Research Group and Transfer Factor from 4Life, which will support the immune system.

To stimulate sec IgA they may suggest taking beta 1–3 glucans, probiotics and *Saccharomyces boulardii*, which is a naturally occurring fungi common to the lychee fruit (see page 68 for more about this).

Managing the gut flora

As described earlier in this chapter, the vital importance of the bacterial colonies that live in the human gut cannot be overstated. The weakened gut defences caused by the depletion of beneficial bacteria through overuse of antibiotics or because of stress, poor diet, and so on, is a hugely significant contributor to leaky gut syndrome, various other malfunctions of the digestive system and an increase in gut-derived toxins; so much so that the function of 'friendly bacteria' has entered the public consciousness. Recent studies by Professor Jeremy Nicholson (head of the department of Surgery and Cancer at Imperial College in London) suggested individuals with an ASC have greater problems dealing with some of these gut-borne toxins released from bad bacteria.

Probiotics and prebiotics: which is which?

To understand how gut flora works you first need to understand the roles and differences between probiotics and prebiotics. Probiotics, in the form of supplements, provide live beneficial bacteria to the gut, and prebiotics are the sugars that feed them to promote colonisation:

Probiotics are commonly dietary supplements containing live bacteria (and sometimes other active microorganisms, such as yeasts).

These probiotic supplements contain specific strains of what are known as 'good bacteria', such as *Lactobacillus* and *Bifidobacteria* in order to recolonise the gut flora, reinforce the immune system and to continue their good work. It is very important to find out which beneficial bacteria are deficient and which pathogenic (or bad) species are active in the gut. There is a simple stool analysis called the comprehensive digestive stool analysis with parasitology that looks at many functions of the gut, including dysbiosis, pH level, digestion and absorption markers.

Prebiotics are non-digestible substances found in some foods that actively 'feed', or stimulate, the growth of good bacteria in the gut.

The two most widely used prebiotics are inulin and fructo-oligosaccharides (FOS). These are carbohydrates (sugars in this case) that occur naturally in a range of foods, the best being those richest in soluble fibre such as Jerusalem artichokes, Brussels sprouts, broccoli, cabbage, onions, leeks, garlic, sweet potatoes, oats, lentils, beans and other pulses, nuts and seeds.

I have had occasional problems in my clinical practice getting beneficial bacteria to thrive in the gut of some individuals, even though 80–120 billion cells have been therapeutically supplemented per day. Beneficial bacteria need 'open' space to colonise; they do not kill off *Candida* and other bacterial species but competitively exclude them by dominating the available space and pushing them out, but only once they have been given the opportunity to occupy the vacant space in the gut. It is important to use a qualified nutritional therapist who is experienced in the specifics of supplementation and also to ensure your child has a diet rich in foods high in soluble fibre.

I always advise parents to think of the gut like a very busy road: the lorries and cars that are parked on the curb-side are the residents (such as the *Candida* and other bacteria species in the gut). Into this environment I introduce a quantity of newer, better cars (probiotics – the beneficial bacteria) that travel along the road looking for spaces, but if there are no spaces to be occupied, then these will just drive on by without parking.

There are a number of influences affecting probiotic colonisation, including acidic pH levels of the gut, a diet lacking in soluble fibre, which is required as a food for the beneficial bacteria, and stomach acid killing off the probiotic bacteria in food supplements before they reach the intestine. It is therefore quite difficult to establish a healthy gut colony of beneficial bacteria if these issues are not addressed prior to using probiotics.

There are also issues with prebiotics, particularly in supplement form. Although naturally occurring prebiotics are effective in 'feeding' good bacteria, there is some debate as to the long-term effects of prebiotic supplements in that they might also feed and encourage the overgrowth of particular types of harmful bacteria.

However, the bottom line has to be that many people benefit from using pro- and prebiotics. Any progress in rebuilding gut flora colonies has to be a good thing in enhancing gut function and boosting the immune system, as well as enhancing digestion and absorption, making nutrients and, above all, reducing toxicity.

Some other dietary recommendations are given below to help support the gut's colony of beneficial bacteria and to reduce the possibility of *Candida* and fungal species occurring:

Reduce consumption of refined carbohydrates. Here's the bad news: refined flour and confectionery – white bread, cakes, biscuits, sweets, and so on – provide exactly the right nutrients (mostly glucose) for *Candida* to thrive on and can upset blood sugar balance. They should be avoided in any attempt to address dysbiosis (see page 49), *Candida* overgrowth and leaky gut syndrome. Other foods suspected to increase *Candida* are cheeses, nuts and seeds, mushrooms, smoked and preserved meats, syrups and honey, dried fruits and citrus fruits, such as oranges and grapefruit.

Anti-fungal foods. The prevalence of *Candida* species has commonly been identified with leaky gut syndrome. Once *Candida* gets a firm hold (commonly associated with dysbiosis and an over-indulgence in refined carbohydrates, fruits and sugar-based foods) they can spread from the gut into the blood system to cause a systemic infection.

Foods such as ginger root, turmeric, garlic, cider vinegar, cloves and oregano, and food and plant compounds such as olive leaf, have been shown to resist fungal overgrowth.

At one time, antibiotic drugs were given with an antifungal agent, so that when the bacteria were destroyed, fungal species were prevented from colonising. The fact that this is no longer common practice may be one of the reasons why *Candida* is now so prevalent in our children. Fungal colonisation can easily lead to increased biofilm production and also to increased gut permeability. Firstly, look for the presence of *Candida* and treat with specific antifungals; your general practitioner may select antifungal drugs such as Nystatin or Diflucan.

I always select the agent that the fungal species is specifically sensitive to, which is commonly berberine, uva ursi, oregano, garlic, capryllic acid or combinations such as Candiclear by Higher Nature or digestive enzymes that breakdown the wall of the *Candida*.

Enzyme food therapy

As far back as the 1950s, Dr Edward Howell discovered that eating plants containing specific digestive enzymes (proteases, lipases, amylases and cellulase) improved the digestion and assimilation of foods. This is important for people with a leaky gut, as the digestion of foods, specifically the breaking down of proteins into their amino-acid form, is important if peptides and polypeptides (for example, the opioid peptides glutamorphin/gliadin and casomorphin) are not to be absorbed through the porous gut membrane.

Basically, it is possible to aid and support the proper digestion of potentially harmful proteins, and to thereby reduce food allergies and support immune function by supplementing the diet with foods rich in the enzymes that the body needs and uses to break them down (catabolise); for example, pineapple and papaya are rich in proteases (bromelain and papain), which are enzymes that break down proteins and peptides into amino acids and are therefore good foods to assist digestion. There are also enzymes which are available as supplements; Houston and Kirkman are two such products, and a qualified nutritionist will be able to advise which ones are appropriate for you.

Individual nutrients and supplements

Apart from pro- and prebiotics there are additional individual supplements that are beneficial for the colonisation and control of gut flora and to support the health of the gut membrane. As before, it is important to consult with a qualified nutritionist before implementing such a regime for your child.

L-Glutamine is an amino acid that is the preferred 'fuel' for the cells in the small intestine. It is also required for the production of intestinal mucus and secretory IgA. It helps to re-establish the protective integrity and digestive function of the gut wall and can help prevent the translocation of bacteria from the gut to the bloodstream.

Butyrate is a short-chain fatty acid that is required as a fuel to support the health of the large intestine. It is produced by beneficial bacteria from the fermentation of soluble fibre.

Vitamin A is also essential for the production of sec IgA. It helps maintain the intestinal mucosa and soothes inflammation.

Vitamin D is essential for the absorption of fats, phosphorus and calcium.

Zinc is extremely important for the maintenance of the intestinal lining. It is required for cell growth and healing, and is essential to cells with a rapid turnover such as those of the small intestine, which are replaced about every 12 days.

N-acetyl cysteine (NAC) is a powerful antioxidant in its own right and is a highly bio-available source of the amino acid cysteine. Cysteine is essential for the production of the body's most useful antioxidant, glutathione. NAC also supports liver function and can support probiotic colonisation, as well as aiding sulphation and is an effective decongestant. It may, however, also support the growth of *Candida* and therefore should not be recommended for individuals with a *Candida* overgrowth.

Saccharomyces boulardii is a non-colonising yeast species that is often included in probiotic treatments. It inhibits the growth and spread of *Candida*, promoting the colonisation of beneficial species such as lactobacilli and *Bifidobacteria*. It also 'switches off' zonulin (a human protein that regulates the permeability of the gut), thereby addressing one of the main culprits in the leaky gut process. *S. boulardii* also aids the digestion of carbohydrates, reducing the wind and bloating that can result if they are not properly digested, and it supports cell re-growth, stimulates sec IgA production and reduces inflammation.

Eliminating a biofilm

Identification of a biofilm is very difficult, although there are a number of likely symptoms for its existence. These can be mucus in the stool, nutrient-deficiency symptoms, a failure to thrive, diarrhoea and/or constipation, odorous stools or undigested food in the stool. The following is therefore seen as a temporary treatment process to support elimination of the biofilm. The biofilm matrix needs to be removed from the system, but this has to be done with great care due to the fact that simply breaking down the structure of the biofilm will release its toxic contents (pathogens, toxins and heavy metals) into the gut, which would be counterproductive. The biofilm utilises metal and mineral compounds (calcium, magnesium and iron) in its structure, so it is not recommended to supplement your diet with these minerals when a biofilm is present.

A number of steps and precautions must be taken to flush out the biofilm: breaking down the fibrin, introducing agents to bind heavy metals and toxins for excretion and supplementing the beneficial gut flora. This is a job for a qualified nutritional therapist.

Improved gut health reaps rewards

There are a number of diagnostic tests available that will enable you, through your practitioner, to identify and treat some of the hidden issues associated with gut function.

Enhancing the health of the gut through a healthy gut membrane, with a lack of biofilm, and with a high production of sec IgA will, in turn, enhance its ability to protect the body from pathogenic and allergenic challenges. The beneficial bacteria will then be able to do their job in supporting nutrient synthesis and availability, because food will be more effectively digested. Nutrient-deficiency symptoms will reduce as nutrient availability and absorption is increased. Healing the gut membrane will reduce allergies and toxins passing to the liver, and this will help to remove the toxic burden on the body.

The significance of good gut health and function is one of the most important areas to address, as individuals with an ASC have many issues associated with poor gut health and function. It should therefore be given priority. In the next chapter I describe further the importance of testing and the journey we made with Billy from taking tests to treating his condition.

CHAPTER 4

From Tests to Treatment and Beyond

During the 12 years, since Billy's diagnosis, through growing research and my clinical experience, I have become more aware of the many underlying issues commonly associated with individuals with an ASC. These may range from gut issues (as explained in Chapter 3), the inability to remove toxins from the body, immune system problems, dietary sensitivities and nutrient deficiencies, as well as heavy metal contamination and many more. It is so difficult, though, to identify these by simply looking at our children on the surface. Some may have eczema, red anal areas, dark eye circles, a pale complexion, rashes or spots on the skin, visible ribs, a poor ability to thrive, and so on, yet the causes of such physical symptoms are rarely addressed by the medical profession. In this chapter I will discuss how diagnostic testing helps us to identify and better understand some of the issues hidden beneath the surface that may well be the cause of our children's diagnoses, and I will also explain how these same issues can be contributory factors to their behaviours, emotions and functional abilities.

The first grains of hope

Recalling Billy's diagnosis and the great pain Polly and I went through to bring ourselves to accept and understand it, still elicits waves of the sadness, hopelessness and the anguish we felt – feelings that only people who have shared that experience could ever understand. We would read stories and reports of autism that painted a very black picture: no friends, no independent life, no love life, no job, no cure, and no hope. The sheer desperation we felt was boundless and almost intolerable. It seemed that no one understood or was ready, or able, to help.

Then someone did offer some help. Not long after Billy was diagnosed – he was two and a half – a concerned neighbour slipped a newspaper cutting through the letterbox about how a diet free of wheat and dairy (gluten and casein) could help children with autism. I wasn't particularly keen, as these foods provide important nutrients, and replacing them in a healthy diet would be tricky. Also, at the time, Billy was subsisting on a none-too-healthy diet that was almost exclusively wheat and dairy – basically wheat biscuits and milk – and he had constant diarrhoea. (We later learned, however, that picky eating may be as a direct result of a food allergy or a deficiency in zinc.) Billy couldn't get enough of the stuff. In spite of this, Polly started baking gluten-free biscuits and buying rice milk to replace cow's milk. (Rice milk is a suitable substitute for cow's milk, as it is easier to digest and less allergenic, and it still provides sufficient nutrition.) Billy didn't take to it immediately of course, and he starved himself for a few days, but then he began to eat the biscuits and drink the rice milk. Within a few days his diarrhoea started to improve. It was still diarrhoea, but much less watery, and we also noticed some improvements in his behaviour.

The results weren't dramatic, but they were significant enough to be noticeable to both of us. They gave me my first inkling that there might be some connection between his constant tummy troubles and his autism, and that we could affect some positive change in Billy by examining his whole health and addressing his diet and his gut issues. A little bit of research put me in touch with an organisation called Allergy Induced Autism (AIA), headed by Rosemary Kessick, and before long we had scraped enough money together for me to fly to the US to attend a conference run by another organisation called Defeat Autism Now (DAN) headed by the Autism Research Institute based in San Diego.

We were excited by the discovery of a whole world of scientists and practitioners who were looking into the biomedical issues that surround autism, and this was the start of my own personal journey towards a better understanding of nutritional science. I already had a thorough grounding in health and fitness, biomechanics and physiology from my degree in Sports Science, and have two brothers and a sister who are doctors, and my mother is a now-retired microbiologist, so I didn't find the biomedical stuff too daunting. I threw myself into further research, eventually took a second degree in nutritional therapy and am now a registered DAN practitioner, running an autism clinic.

Of course, although Billy's chronic symptoms had improved on the GFCF diet, his overall health, behaviour and development continued to trouble us deeply and things were still pretty bad.

The only way forward was to do whatever we could to give Billy the best possible opportunities in life, to continue to look into any ways we could find that might possibly help, and to continue to lavish him with love, enthusiasm, support and encouragement.

Then I heard about something that had happened in the US, and Polly and I leapt at what seemed like the first real morsel of hope we'd been offered since the whole nightmare had begun.

The secretin story

In 1998 an American couple named Gary and Victoria Beck hit the headlines in the US when they arranged for their three-year-old son with autism, Parker, to have the hormone secretin administered as a therapy for his autism. Importantly, they had seen amazing results.

This had come about because several of Mrs Beck's relatives had suffered from gastrointestinal disorders and had undergone a diagnostic test known as a 'secretin challenge test'. As Parker also had recurrent gastrointestinal problems, Mrs Beck requested this test for him.

The test examines the health and function of the pancreas by stimulating it with secretin. This naturally occurring hormone of the digestive system is normally secreted by cells in the lining of the duodenum in order to stimulate the pancreas into producing pancreatic juices. These juices are vital to digestion.

Following this relatively routine test using secretin, Parker Beck made what appeared to be a dramatic recovery. His persistent diarrhoea, eye-contact problems, lack of spoken language, difficult behaviour and social skills all improved within weeks, leading the Becks (after further investigation) to seek further doses of secretin.

Parker's combination of autism and gastrointestinal problems rang all sorts of bells with us, and the reported outcomes of his treatment were truly impressive. We felt we had nothing to lose, so we pursued this line of enquiry with renewed vigour. With invaluable help from my contacts in the US we eventually found a way to get hold of secretin and found a doctor who was willing to undertake the procedure in the UK.

Things start to change

Billy's response to the treatment was very encouraging, and following his injections we saw a dramatic change in our son: his eye contact was better, his tummy was less swollen, there were improvements in his concentration, alertness, attention and sociability – and he had his first decent, massive, solid stool (not diarrhoea) in 18 months! Best of all, Billy started to vocalise, not much, but something we thought we would never hear – his voice.

We were delighted with the outcomes, and because Billy was the first child in the UK to undergo this treatment, we found ourselves and our family in the media spotlight. Excited at the time by what appeared to be a major breakthrough in Billy's treatment for his health issues, we were happy to go along with the media interest, including allowing a film crew to accompany us for the secretin treatments and telling 'Billy's Story' to Trevor McDonald on national television in his *Tonight with Trevor McDonald* programme screened at the end of April 1999.

Following the screening of this programme, we were inundated with thousands of calls and emails from other utterly desperate parents with questions, concerns and their own stories, particularly about how difficult it was to find information about resources, interventions and therapies available to help their children with autism.

It was this ongoing clamour for help and support that led Polly to set up the *Autism File* magazine later that year.

Looking deeper

Billy had six secretin infusions between November 1998 and September 1999, but by this stage I was already becoming a little sceptical. It's not that secretin wasn't helping; far from it, we had already seen significant improvements and many (although by no means all) parents had started to get similar results. It was just that it occurred to me that Billy should be making his own secretin. Getting to the bottom of why this naturally occurring hormone was lacking in Billy seemed to be more important and potentially more helpful than just topping it up.

When all was said and done, our little Billy wasn't cured; he still had autism, albeit 'less so'. There were noticeable improvements in lots of areas, but I felt we needed more answers. I started by asking myself a number of questions: why had secretin had such positive effects on Billy? What does secretin actually do? Why was Billy's own ability to produce secretin impaired? Does this indicate a gut-related disorder at the root of Billy's autism? This was the start of a massive quest for information and answers that introduced me to a network of fabulous people and dedicated organisations all over the world, all battling with similar questions.

So, secretin had been beneficial, but it wasn't 'the answer'; more like part of the question, and I therefore stopped the treatment.

However, having been encouraged by our first significant foray into the world of possibilities offered by biomedical interventions, I was more intent than ever on finding out what was going on inside Billy. I knew that further investigation and more serious attention to alleviating the devastating effects of his health issues would be involved – medical testing and possibly additional treatments as well as specific educational requirements, changes to domestic arrangements, and so on – but there now seemed to be a glimmer of light at the end of the tunnel.

My investigations continued

We were convinced by this stage that Billy's descent into autism was directly connected to his physical health and medical history, his immune system and the overuse of antibiotics, his recurrent chest and ear infections, his allergic reactions to milk and wheat and his sudden and violent reaction to the MMR jab.

A picture was starting to emerge, but there were still many pieces missing. The specific metabolic mechanisms at play were still a mystery. I had to know more about how all these and other factors had 'set him up' to trigger autism.

I began to research tests that would enable us to look more closely at the functioning of Billy's immune and digestive systems. There were many of them: food allergies; levels of harmful bacterial (such as Clostridia) and fungal pathogens (like *Candida*) in his gut; liver function and the ability to detoxify; heavy-metal contamination; sec IgA antibody production; vitamin and mineral deficiencies; and so on. I looked into anything that was available or that we could think of to try to pin down what had happened and what we might be able to do about it. I felt we were on to something, and I couldn't see any downside to pursuing every possible thread.

Over the next few months I initiated a range of diagnostic tests and delved into my own and our family's medical histories in order to piece the puzzle together.

Family history is the place to start

If there's one thing that the scientific community can agree on in relation to the aetiology (the origin or cause) of autism, it's that there is a genetic component, a genetic propensity that is passed down through families. If you are somewhere on the autistic continuum, you are more likely to have a child who develops autism, and if you already have one child who develops autism, you are more likely to have another. While the chance that a first child will have autism is about 1 in 100, the chance that a sibling of a child with autism will also have autism is as high as 1 in 5 ('Early Autism Diagnosis: The Infant Sibling Study' by Kimberley Crandell). The same is of course true with a range of other illnesses and disorders. If you have a family history of arthritis, immune-system disorders, mental disorders, heart disease, cancer and allergies, to name but a few – the likelihood of you or your children suffering similar illnesses is automatically higher.

I believe that Billy's descent into autism was caused by a particular combination of circumstances: from a genetic predisposition and a range of environmental and medical factors which suppressed his immune system and triggered a biochemical domino effect that adversely affected his body and brain and eventually flicked the final switch into autism. Clearly the switch had to be there, and clearly all the relevant (genetic) connections beneath the switch had to be in place.

Our contention is that many children inherit and carry this configuration of 'wiring', but its potential is only realised by making further connections and flicking certain switches.

It is very evident from the research that has been completed that individuals with an ASC do not function on a biological level as well as individuals who are 'neurotypical'.

Look beneath the surface: most, if not all biological issues associated with autism can be identified and supported by nutritional and dietary therapies, and with this in mind the use of diagnostic testing is imperative. It is not possible to know the underlying issues to this condition unless you find them through testing. As an example depression is caused predominantly by a low level of serotonin, so to help alleviate depression the cause needs to be addressed, such as identifying why serotonin levels are low. The cause may be insufficient dietary intake of tryptophan or because of inflammatory actions within the body, which means that the conversion of tryptophan to serotonin is reduced as a direct result. Other causes may be low levels of the amino acid isoleucine, or mercury toxicity may be high in the body and essential fatty acids may be low. The goal is to find the cause of the symptom and to address it and not just to aim to treat the symptom with drugs.

When dealing and treating individuals with an ASC it is very important to do just that, and there are many questions you have to ask: how do I know how well my child can get rid of toxins in the body? How do I know what is causing their gut disturbances? How do I know how well they are digesting foods and absorbing nutrients? How do I know what pathogenic infection they may be carrying? These simple questions have answers. The detailed approach to finding out the causative issues to their symptoms must be identified if the correct interventions, and the specific interventions based upon the needs of the individual, are to be addressed.

Why test?

It is regrettable that so many paediatricians, doctors and other healthcare professionals, who are there to look after our children, know so very little about the issues affecting them, and therefore many parents are left to struggle on alone without direction and support. This is a very real, very common and very tragic situation. Our children are shrouded in illness and dysfunction and we have to get to the root of it.

Think of your child's illness as a multi-layered cocoon. Each layer of toxicity and dysfunction has to be stripped away and the next layer revealed, like a deeply serious game of 'pass the parcel', with your healthy child as the prize within. The layers of illness might be due to inflammation, heavy-metal toxicity, free-radical damage, bacterial, viral, fungal or parasitic overgrowth or infection, glandular dysfunction, hormonal imbalance, immuno-suppression, allergy or intolerance, and so on. Your child cannot break out of these layers, so we as parents, supported by the relevant professionals, have to break in. We have to identify, treat and eradicate each layer, and this starts with diagnostic testing.

Laboratory testing uses scientific analysis to pinpoint issues that may be relevant to the health and well-being of a particular individual. The results of these tests help to establish a specific treatment protocol with the overall aim of correcting abnormalities and restoring optimal health and functioning.

In recent years there has been a significant shift in the type of treatment protocols offered by practitioners to treat health disorders. With this comes a better understanding and usage of diagnostic tests performed by clinical laboratories worldwide.

Functional biomedical testing evaluates how well various organs and body systems are performing, and can include metabolic, digestive, nutritional and immunological assessment, through to detoxification, endocrine and exocrine (glandular) hormonal balances and allergenic and toxicity profiles.

These types of assessment enable a greater insight into the many variable processes that may lead to the acquisition of illness and diseases (aetiology). This is especially true when dealing with individuals with autism, due to the high prevalence of gastrointestinal, immunological and toxicity issues in this group.

Where pinpointing the problems begins

In my clinical practice, I have found it important to use the tests available through a select group of laboratories recognised for their abilities to reproduce tests of the highest standard; testing in those organisations is stringently controlled to protect against human and technological error. These labs offer a professional service and provide practitioners with support in interpreting the results. They also have an ongoing interest in laboratory development and research.

Before I undertake any testing through The Autism Clinic I ask parents to complete a specially devised questionnaire in as much detail and as accurately as possible, and to provide all previous reports and test results they may already have. This detail on medical history, family history, symptoms and sensitivities enables me to build up a picture of the child before seeing him or her in the clinic and it gives me a starting point for my investigations. The questionnaire is available to download via www.theautismclinic.com.

Identifying the health symptoms will determine where further investigations should take you. With the guidance of a qualified and experienced professional, you can begin to understand the layers of illness that affect your child and then begin to put in place measures to address them by using treatment protocols specifically designed for your child.

Having now had much experience in dealing with autism, not only through Billy but the numerous clinic patients I see, the main areas requiring further investigations via diagnostic testing need to focus on gut function, detoxification impairments and immune dysfunction, which leads to impaired brain function. This is vitally important for you when finding out through your qualified practitioner what is wrong with your child, and through thorough investigation it will enable a specific treatment protocol to be designed, enabling you to look forward to some positive results and achievements.

Billy's tests and treatment

We conducted a number of initial tests on Billy when he was about three years seven months old, with the hope of developing a greater awareness, understanding and appreciation of his state of health. All the tests we undertook opened new avenues for us to follow in our quest to find solutions to the puzzle of autism.

We took hair, blood, urine and stool samples, and sent them off for laboratory analysis. The results showed significant issues that needed to be addressed.

In the course of this initial foray into biomedical testing I uncovered evidence of active measles infection and parasites in the gut, an imbalance of gut flora and an overgrowth of pathogenic species. I also found Billy exhibited allergies to a range of foods as well as having a recent infection due to glandular fever, a number of inherited or acquired toxins, digestive enzyme deficiencies and malabsorption of nutrients. These illnesses and dysfunctions helped to form the multi-layered cocoon that had engulfed my son.

I understood then that until these burdens were identified and addressed, Billy would not be able to reverse his health issues. Treating the many issues we found allowed the return of a normally functioning gut and improved immunity so that Billy was better able to detoxify and neutralise freely.

This is not an easy task for anyone, and I was assisted by many professionals around the world who read through the results of Billy's various tests and suggested the direction for treatment. Based on their advice, and using my own knowledge, I was able to cross-refer their suggestions and formulate an effective plan of action. Those professionals helped me to pave the way to a brighter future for my son.

Billy's treatment protocol

Based upon Billy's symptoms and results, and their interpretation, the initial treatment was an extensive protocol using a selected range of organic, hypo-allergenic foods and nutritional and supportive supplements. These ranged from enzymes, coconut oil, an anti-virus supplement (Monolaurin), probiotics, gut-restoring amino acids, essential fatty acids, antioxidants and detoxification support, immune modulators and enhancers through to heavy-metal clathration products and vitamins, minerals, trace elements and amino acids. Remember that this supplemental protocol, which was individual to Billy only, was completed following months of diagnostic testing and after seeking advice from numerous experts. Of course, the range of treatments were specific to his case, and it is never appropriate to try a variety of treatments without specialist help. I'm giving you the details here only so that you can better understand what effective treatment of your child might involve.

I clearly remember how difficult it was trying to get Billy to swallow this quantity of daily supplements. The only way we could manage it in the early days was by mixing ground-up tablets, tinctures and powders with sugar-free maple syrup. He still wasn't at all happy about taking the mixture, though.

Over the years Billy's protocols have changed many times as updated test results have shown us where he has improved and which areas still needed addressing.

Happily, he will now voluntarily swallow capsules and tablets, and washes them down with water.

Help from a special diet

Billy was put on a strict GFCF diet and I also focused on introducing new whole foods that were rich in those nutrients he was deficient in. I also included foods high in soluble fibre – such as Brussels sprouts, cabbage, onions, Jerusalem artichokes and garlic – to support his beneficial gut bacteria. All the foods he consumed were organic and free from additives and preservatives. We also gave him exclusively filtered water to drink. (In Chapter 10 I discuss suitable diets for children with autism.)

Reassuring improvements

Billy is in good health with no abnormal intestinal permeability, a good gut flora balance and no need for additional antioxidants, minerals or trace elements. He now enjoys a very diverse range of foods, and no longer needs to keep his diet gluten- and casein-free, which he now digests and absorbs well.

Not a bad result, considering his initial diagnosis: a diagnosis that we were told he would always have, a condition we could do nothing about; and we would have to face the fact that our son would end up in an institution. I do hope that many of you reading this book, with a child who has an ASC, will not be blinkered by the information you are given by those who know very little about nutritional interventions that can help our children.

Having now worked with more than 500 individuals diagnosed with an ASC, I have yet to find a single child who is in perfect health; however, through correctly identifying the many hidden issues that commonly affect our children's functioning, and by using specific treatments available today, we can pave the way to a much brighter future for them. As a parent of a child with autism, you have a long journey ahead of you, but please persevere – find the right practitioner with the knowledge, experience and professionalism who will support you.

Remember, autism is a psychologically diagnosed condition with an underlying biological cause.

In the next chapter I explore the role that toxins play in the development of autism.

CHAPTER 5

The Link with Toxins

People often say to me that autism is a purely genetic condition, and this also seems to be the general consensus of mainstream medical science. Some parents say that their child was 'born autistic' and for some that may well be the case, but evidence I have gathered from my clinical questionnaire, of which 200 of the 500 responses have so far been statistically evaluated, shows that only 1 per cent of children attending my clinic with an ASC are thought by their parents to have been born autistic. Sixty-four per cent cite a suspected delay from between 6 and 18 months, and 76 per cent of those gradually regressed into an autistic condition. Forty per cent of respondents state that their child lost spoken words (the language they had previously) between 12 and 18 months.

The vast majority of parents whose children I have seen in my clinic believe that autism 'happened' to their child at some stage in their early years.

The first links between the environment and autism

Leo Kanner, the psychiatrist at Johns Hopkins University who first identified autism from his study on 11 children back in 1943, found that, aside from his diagnostic criteria for autism, many exhibited clear indications of a regressive condition. He wrote the following in separate case reports:

> The mother, in commenting on Richard's failure to talk, remarked in her notes – 'I can't be sure when he stopped the imitation of word sounds, it seems that he has gone backwards mentally gradually for the last two years.'

> Seemed alert and responsive as an infant and said many words at eighteen months, but toward the end of the second year she did not show much progression in her play relationships or in contacts with other people.

> Normal birth, she appeared healthy, took feeding well, stood up at seven months and walked at less than a year. She could say a few words at the end of her first year but made no progress in linguistic development for the following four years.

Kanner also identified biomedical, gastrointestinal and immunological issues in these children:

> He was born normally. He vomited a great deal during his first year and feeding formulas were changed frequently with little success. His tonsils were removed when he was three years old.

> He suffered from repeated colds and Otitis Media which necessitated bilateral myringotomy [incision in the ear drum, often with grommets inserted].

So, back then, the issues of regression into an autistic state and the association with biomedical conditions were evident. Again and again research studies have shown abnormalities in respect to immunology, detoxification, gastrointestinal disturbances and their interrelationships with aberrant brain function. There are also studies pointing to associated inherited genetic-coding problems relating to impaired abilities to get rid of toxins.

A susceptibility to developing autism

My conclusion has to be that autism is a predisposed, regressive disorder; that is, autism is predisposed in some people owing to factors carried in their genes, but that these 'markers', or aberrant genes, need to be 'switched on' by environmental factors in order for autism to be activated. Just taken purely objectively, the difference in the pattern of the onset and characteristics of an ASC must surely indicate a range of variables in the reasons for its causes, as is stated here: 'Data suggests that autism results from multiple etiologies with both genetic and environmental contributions, which may explain the spectrum of behaviors seen in this disorder.' (Libbey, et al., 'Autistic disorder and viral infections', *Journal of Neurovirology*, vol. 11, No. 1 (2005):1–10).

It is clear and incontestable that there is a genetic component to the susceptibility to autism, but all the available evidence points to the fact that carrying the 'susceptibility gene' for autism (if there is such a thing – we await the best efforts of geneticists), indicates a predisposition, not a fait accompli. In other words, it's possible to avoid flicking the switch, or at least to turn the dimmer down to its lowest setting. I'm by no means alone in believing that environmental factors contribute to the onset of autism, and there is a great deal of interest and academic research worldwide into a huge variety of factors that might contribute. As discussed by Dr Robert Bransfield MD at the Autism 1 Conference in Chicago in 2008, human illness and disease is commonly caused by the individual having susceptible genes that, if challenged by environmental insults, will lead to dysfunction, infection and disease. Autism may have many susceptible genes that can be altered in the way they work by toxins, heavy metals, nutrient deficiencies and vaccination. This then may impact on the health of the individual, their immune system, their ability to detoxify and the way in which their brain functions.

The environmental factor

Environmental toxicity has changed since the Industrial Revolution, and the growing list of foreign chemicals or toxins we are exposed to in our contemporary society is simply outrageous. Every ocean, every continent and every natural habitat, from the tropics to the polar regions, is now contaminated.

So, is this the reason why autism rates have risen so dramatically over the past 30 years? Before the 1990s, it was estimated that approximately four children in every 10,000 (1 in 2,500) had autism in the UK. Now, a shocking new statistic from the Cambridge Research Institute has shown that autism may affect as many as 1 in 64 children. That's 156 in every 10,000.

Many experts will tell you that ASCs were poorly recognised and under-diagnosed in the 1980s and that the perceived increase is a result of improved diagnosis, increased awareness and broadening of diagnostic criteria, and while this is likely to be true to some extent, it cannot account for such a massive, exponential increase. There are clearly other factors at play here.

As I've previously said, there are undoubtedly genetic factors involved in the aetiology of autism, but this doesn't help at all in understanding why rates of the condition are soaring. You can't have a genetic epidemic.

When detoxification becomes faulty

My understanding is that the predisposition for autism exists on an immunological level and that whether the switch is flicked on or not depends on how a genetically impaired immune system copes with gut inflammation and reduced natural detoxification abilities due to impairments in detoxification.

These impairments in vital metabolic functions will leave

an infant susceptible to inflammation caused by pathogenic opportunists (bacteria, viruses, yeasts and the like) and allergens, as well as to environmental toxins and a cascade of genetic and cellular damage and dysfunction.

The gastrointestinal (GI) tract contains the largest immune-active tissue in the body, as it is the site with the greatest exposure to pathogens and toxins. Toxins pass through the gut wall into the portal vein and are delivered to the liver for neutralisation and elimination. Most detoxification then occurs in the liver, where the liver cells (hepatocytes) modify toxins so that they can be excreted or eliminated from the body.

Toxins ingested in our food, inhaled from the atmosphere or released as by-products of bacterial, viral or fungal activity, and so on, can build up in the body and cause untold damage to various organs and systems. The liver has incredibly sophisticated mechanisms for dealing with many of these (more on this remarkable organ later), but it can only do so much, and can either fail to do it due to its own dysfunction or can be overwhelmed by the sheer volume or potency of the toxins.

But how do these toxins manage to affect brain functioning?

Toxins and the brain

In some cases, toxins that make it through the body's defences can have access to the brain and central nervous system (CNS), directly affecting different types of neurons either by attacking the nerve cells or by interfering with the electrical impulses, which then affect the signals received by the brain. What is not well known, however, is that the gut has its own brain: the enteric nervous system (ENS – often called the 'second brain'). The neurons in the ENS control 'mechanical' functions of the gut, such as the secretion of digestive enzymes and the muscular contractions of peristalsis (see page 46) and emotional responses such as 'butterflies in the stomach' and fear-induced diarrhoea. These reactions result from the sensory neurons in the gut reacting to the release of 'fight or flight' hormones such as adrenalin, and to the increased production of the neurotransmitter serotonin, which is abundant in the gut and has a major role in controlling peristalsis and the speed of bowel movements.

The blood–brain barrier

The structural lining surrounding the brain – the blood–brain barrier – is designed to prevent toxins from reaching and damaging important neurons, in much the same way as the gut membrane is designed to prevent the passage of certain molecules and microbes into the bloodstream. Clearly, this barrier has to be permeable to allow the passage of essential nutrients, so it can be crossed, and indeed some modern medicines and drugs are designed to do so in order to have a desired effect on brain functioning.

The blood–brain barrier is not fully formed in infants, and research is starting to show that it may not be fully formed until much later, possibly well into adolescence. This may then enable unwanted toxins to pass into the brain structure and alter the way in which it functions; however, the actual mechanisms that regulate the two-way flow of information between the ENS and the brain are not fully understood, neither is the complex interplay between various toxins and the blood–brain barrier. What we do know is that the vagus nerve can transport toxins directly from the gut to the brain.

Where do toxins come from?

Toxins are derived from numerous sources, and can have dramatic effects on the body: some are the chemicals or bi-products of chemicals that are part of the food we eat, either occurring naturally or added during food production; some are the waste products of our own metabolism; some are produced by the 'bad guys' living in the gut; some are the result of the defensive reactions of our own immune system, killing off microbes it destroys; and some are the woeful consequence of decades of heavy industry, medicinal pharmaceuticals and chemicals that are in the air that we breathe, the food that we eat, the domestic products that we use every day and in the soil beneath our feet. Research on umbilical-cord blood from newborn babies has identified almost 300 toxic chemicals in its composition. These chemicals are all foreign to our bodies and therefore require detoxification to remove them. The complex dance of detoxification that our bodies have to undergo involves the neutralisation and elimination of all foreign toxins unwanted for human health.

Biotoxins and neurotoxins

Detoxification problems associated with an ASC have led to a number of studies looking at the role of biotoxins in relation to neurological disturbances. Biotoxins include microbial toxins derived from organisms residing within the human body, such as bacteria, viruses, parasites, fungi and yeasts.

Toxins that have a direct effect on the nerve cells (neurons) of the brain or nervous system are called neurotoxins. Neurotoxins are attracted to the nervous system. They are taken in by nerve endings and disrupt vital functions of the nerve cells, such as nutrient transport, production of energy and gene expression (the way in which our genes and their DNA codes actually work).

Neurotoxins, in order of toxicity, include:

- Heavy metals, such as tin, mercury, aluminium, cadmium, antimony, lead, arsenic and fluorine.
- Biotoxins and microbial toxins released by bacteria, such as tetanus, botulinum and proprionic acid.
- Inflammatory toxins, such as nitric oxide, quinolinic acid and peroxynitrite.
- Mycotoxins from fungal species.

- Xenobiotics (man-made environmental toxins, such as dioxin, phthalates, formaldehyde, insecticides and pesticides, wood preservatives, and so on).
- Food additives and preservatives, such as aspartame and monosodium glutamate, and so on.

The body finds neurotoxins more difficult to eradicate than other pathogens because of their specialised ability to invade and disrupt nerve cells, and many are absorbed by the abundant nerve endings found in the enteric nervous system of the gut wall. Neurotoxins are lipophilic (fat-liking), which means that they can be dissolved in fat and are attracted to structures that are rich in fat, especially the cells found in the gut, liver, kidney and brain.

Children with autism who have attended my clinic have undergone a test called organic acid analysis or the Optimal Nutrition Evaluation tests, and I have found that many show clear dysfunctions in mitochondrial energy production due to heavy metal toxicity and nutrient deficiency. Mitochondria are the self-contained structures (organelles) within cells that are responsible for generating energy from our food, and dysfunction in this process can lead to early cell death and generally poor metabolism.

With our current chemical burden, our bodies are constantly under stress and an enormous toxic load. My argument here is that children who go on to develop autism have the same exposure to vaccinations, environmental toxins and heavy metals as all other children, but the problem lies with how our children cannot cope, owing to genetic predispositions or changes to their genes as a result of poor detoxification.

We know that in order for the gut to be protected, an appropriate immune response is required to prevent damage from the bad guys and food allergens. A distorted immune system, poor at protecting the gut, leads to an imbalance in gut flora, which in turn progresses to inflammation and damage. This suppresses the main antioxidant, glutathione, and increases the permeability of both the blood–brain barrier and the gut. Greater levels of toxins, food allergens and pathogens can therefore pass through the gut membrane into the blood system putting stress on the liver, the immune system and all detoxification systems.

Cleansing the system through detoxification

Detoxification is highly important for all people with autism, especially, as many have nutrient deficiencies, heavy metal burdens, poor methylation, sulphation and a toxic load exacerbated by ever increasing environmental sources. As we have seen, natural detoxification can be weakened and impaired in many ways in individuals with an ASC, so this vital process needs to be supported.

Detoxification is all about how the body gets rid of toxins (foreign substances), or unstable molecules, caused by oxidation, that together cause damage to the cell, its contents and its function. It is vital that nutrients and antioxidants that support toxin neutralisation and removal are available in good amounts and that the liver and other organs responsible for excreting toxins are functioning optimally.

The liver is the body's most important organ for eliminating these toxins, ably aided by the body's most potent antioxidant, glutathione.

The multifunctional liver

The liver serves many vital functions in the body (more than 500 individual processes), particularly in killing microbes, supporting metabolism, processing nutrients, making hormones and neurotransmitters, filtering toxins from the blood, producing bile to help break down fats, and storing various vitamins and minerals.

The detoxification abilities of the liver are vital to health and well-being, and any impairment can have significant effects. If pushed too hard, symptoms of liver stress will appear:

- Lethargy and decreased energy
- Increased allergic reactions
- Brain fog
- Poor memory and concentration
- Mood swings
- Depression
- Coated tongue (*Candida*)
- Bad breath
- Dark eye circles
- Pale coloured stools
- Stools that float
- Erratic blood sugar control
- Abdominal weight gain
- Fat deposits beneath the skin

If your child experiences any of these symptoms, then liver stress and issues related to detoxification are certainly worth consideration, especially as many autistic individuals have an increased susceptibility towards poor detoxification. The liver is an organ that is not often discussed in the field of autism, but I personally feel that it is heavily associated with many of the issues associated with the condition, including the following disturbances found commonly in people with autism:

- Poor ability to detoxify
- Methylation and sulphation problems
- High general toxicity levels
- Leaky gut – increasing absorption of toxins, allergens and pathogens
- Hormone imbalances: insulin, adrenalin, cortisol and serotonin

- Poor digestion of fats
- Candidiasis and constipation
- Low levels of beneficial gut flora
- pH imbalance in the gut
- Increased food allergens
- Low levels of B vitamins, especially B_6 and B_{12}
- Vitamin D and mineral deficiencies
- Poor liver enzyme function
- Heavy metal toxicity

I have seen many children in my clinic with chronic dysbiosis, permeability of the gut membrane, constipation and other gut issues that enhance and exacerbate toxin production and re-sorption. Remember that all toxins are passed via the GI tract into the portal vein and carried to the liver for nutrient processing and toxin elimination. If your child has the disturbances listed above, then there will be an increased exposure to toxins, and an inability to detoxify naturally. These are all common issues and therefore need to be addressed.

Excretion

Much of the detoxification function of the liver relies on other essential bodily processes to rid the body of toxins and their components once they've been neutralised or broken down. These functions are known collectively as 'excretion' and this occurs through five methods of elimination:

1. Urine
2. Faeces
3. Sweat
4. Hair
5. Breath

These obviously need to be functioning well if the final elimination of toxins is to happen efficiently.

Urine: the function of the kidneys is to filter the blood and prepare toxic substances for evacuation. Under normal circumstances, the kidneys are incredibly efficient at filtering out virtually everything from the blood as well as regulating the body's salt and water content, but they need a regular intake of fluids to do this. Many people with autism do not drink enough fluids or eat enough foods with a high water content, such as fruit and vegetables. Because it is important to urinate regularly so that toxins can be eliminated, keeping your child well hydrated is imperative.

Faeces: the end waste product of the digestive system can be remarkably informative in identifying digestive issues, as I explained on page 51. Gastrointestinal issues commonly affect people with autism and impact on their ability to eliminate toxins, especially if constipation is an issue.

When the gut is not functioning well and is in poor health its ability to eliminate the toxins is impaired. Indeed, more toxins are produced caused by fermentation, putrefaction and an increase in time exposed to these in the gut. Leaky gut (page 57) will also increase the levels of toxic resorption, and impaired liver function reduces elimination.

Sweat rids the body of various waste substances including salts (sodium, chloride and potassium), uric acid, lactic acid, ammonia and tiny amounts of various minerals, including toxic metals. For centuries, saunas and steam therapy have been used to initiate sweating to aid detoxification, and exercise will serve much the same purpose.

Hair: any substance, including toxins, which can circulate in the bloodstream, can be deposited where capillaries carry blood supply to the hair follicles. There is an ongoing debate about traces of heavy metals, particularly mercury, which are detectable in hair samples, because some children with autism show significant traces of mercury whereas others do not. The excretion of mercury detectible in hair clearly indicates that there is some ability to remove this toxin from the body, whereas many people with autism have deficiencies in the heavy-metal transporters, called metallothionein proteins, which reduce their ability to transport heavy metals to the hair follicle. As a consequence those people may be extremely toxic in heavy metals.

Breath is another way in which the body excretes waste products such as methane, ethanol, carbon dioxide and hydrogen. It can be measured to assess bacterial and fungal overgrowth in the gut.

Removing heavy metals

On page 89 we discussed the issue of toxic heavy metals (especially mercury, but also others including arsenic, tin, aluminium, cadmium and lead) and the problems they can cause. Reduced levels of glutathione and metallothionein can substantially impair the body's natural ability to rid the system of these poisons, but removing them is essential. Heavy-metal chelation therapy uses chemical agents such as EDTA, DMPS or DMSA (prescribed only by a medical professional) to bond to heavy metals in the system and prepare them for excretion, but this can be quite an invasive, expensive and potentially dangerous process, so please seek advice from a qualified chelation expert before embarking on this issue. Furthermore, chelation therapy will reduce beneficial elements, such as zinc, selenium, copper, magnesium and calcium, so it is imperative that a suitably qualified practitioner is consulted. Fundamental tests, such as the hair mineral analysis by Doctor's Data labs, urinary porphyrins from Philippe Auguste Laboratoire and the Optimal Nutrition Evaluation profile from Genova Diagnostics laboratory may show some heavy-metal toxicity, but remember that these elevations or normal readings in both hair and urine may not represent the complete picture, as your qualified therapist will be aware.

Clathration

Rather than chemical chelation, I use a slower and much safer option called 'clathration', utilising the natural properties of chlorella (algae), cilantro (coriander) and alpha-lipoic acid (a natural antioxidant).

Chlorella vulgaris is a whole food and a complete protein that binds to toxins for excretion. It also has the ability to reactivate the body's detoxification functions as well as increasing glutathione and helping to support metallothionein production. It also contains amino acids, beta-carotene, minerals and vitamins B_{12} and B_6, and it helps restore gut bacteria levels and reduces acidosis.

Cilantro has the effect of 'mobilising' heavy metal toxins, such as nickel, cadmium, aluminium, lead and mercury. It dislocates these toxic molecules from their hiding places in intracellular spaces so that they can be effectively excreted. (Because it does this, it is important to combine its use with *Chlorella vulgaris*.) This is a safer option, in my opinion, and one that is less likely to create resorption issues of heavy metals 'freed' from their hiding place and released into the blood system ready for excretion from the body.

Alpha-lipoic acid is a natural antioxidant, very effective in eliminating heavy metals.

I also use other supportive nutrients, such as selenium, glutathione, zinc, magnesium, calcium and cysteine. A qualified nutritionist experienced in heavy-metal detoxification can help you with this, if heavy metals are an issue.

The role of glutathione

As I've pointed out on many occasions, glutathione is the most prevalent and potent antioxidant and detoxifier a body could wish for. It is found in every cell and is vital to protect the cells from damage. A significant deficiency in glutathione is common in people with autism and is increasingly being viewed and researched as a major factor in the condition.

Oxidative stress to cells can damage energy-generating mitochondria and it can alter the composition of cell membranes and essential proteins. It can also disrupt DNA. This in turn can lead to abnormal gene expression and impairments in neural development and signal transmission (including nerve cells and neural pathways).

Glutathione is synthesised in the body from the three amino acids, cysteine, glycine and glutamate, with the sulphurous element of cysteine being the main 'active ingredient'. This complete process is a complex sequence of steps known as methylation and transulphation which are dependent on a balance of critical enzymes and nutrients such as vitamins B_{12} and B_6, magnesium, S-adenosylmethionine (SAMe), betaine, potassium, folic acid, sulphate and the amino acids methionine, cysteine, glycine and glutamine.

The key point here is that these pathways have been found to be disrupted in autism by deficiencies or imbalances in many of the essential nutrients, and this is why oxidative stress, toxic burden and heavy-metal contamination are prevalent in individuals with an ASC.

Helping the liver to detoxify

There is overwhelming evidence that doing whatever we can to reduce the exposure to toxins, and supporting the liver in its detoxification functions, is a fundamental part of improving the health of individuals with autism, and it may also bring about dramatic changes in behaviour, mood and ability.

If you provide the vital and necessary nutrients required by the liver to function, you will enable your child to detoxify more efficiently and this will take the stress off the liver. Helping the liver to detoxify should be given priority alongside correcting gut issues, addressing adrenal function, restoring immune function and reducing inflammation, as already discussed.

As explained earlier, many toxins and most neurotoxins are fat loving and fat soluble, and are readily stored in fat tissue, which makes them harder to eliminate than other pathogens. The liver has a method of getting rid of them by using a system of strong enzymes that takes the toxin from being fat soluble and converts them into a water-soluble toxin ready to be excreted.

Supporting the liver nutritionally

Help the liver to detoxify by following the diet suggestions below:

- Cut out all refined carbohydrates and sugar.
- Cut out saturated, trans- and hydrogenated fats (fats hold on to toxins and make the liver sluggish).
- Increase water – drink at least 1 litre (1¾ pints) per day, preferably of purified water (see page 100). (These quantities are suitable for both children and teenagers.)
- Increase those vegetables, seeds and nuts that support the liver: garlic, Jerusalem artichokes, leeks, onions, Brussels sprouts, broccoli, parsley, beetroot, radish, cabbage, spring greens, kale, dandelion, watercress, sesame seeds and walnuts.
- Increase the following fruits: apricot, avocado, banana, blackberries, blueberries, strawberries, raspberries, cranberries, pomegranate, lemon, papaya, pineapple, watermelon, tomatoes and tangerine.
- Increase foods with sulphur-containing amino acids (cysteine, methionine and taurine): sunflower and sesame seeds, oats, Brazil nuts, eggs, fish, meat and organ meats.
- Eat liver and red meat (for three meals per week) for the carnitine contained therein, which pushes fat into cells to

be burned as fuel and therefore reduces the opportunity for toxic storage.

- Drink dandelion tea and tinctures, lemon and green tea.

The following beneficial herbs also support the liver, but must be prescribed by a qualified herbalist:

- Blackroot, burdock, nettle and bog bean help to prevent constipation.
- Dandelion triggers the contraction of the gall bladder, and thereby increases bile flow and increases liver repair.
- Milk thistle, or silymarin, stimulates gall bladder and bile flow, and may aid liver repair.
- Turmeric is a potent anti-inflammatory herb, which stimulates the gall bladder and bile flow, and may aid in increasing stomach acid secretions.

Avoid toxic chemicals

As well as supporting the body's natural ability to eliminate toxins you also need to reduce the toxins your child is continuously exposed to. Consider reducing all toxins from environmental, dietary and household sources. It's virtually impossible to avoid all environmental toxins but you can try some or all of the following to cut down your exposure:

- Eat organic produce and free-range, organic foods rather than pesticide-controlled or processed foods.
- Seek natural brands of toiletries and cosmetics. Avoid cosmetic products such as soaps, toothpaste and deodorants containing triclosan (which is a chlorophenol, suspected of causing cancer).
- Use biodegradable products wherever possible; for example, Ecover washing liquid and laundry detergent, Ecoballs or soap nuts to wash clothing.

- Avoid eating even moderate-risk fish, such as tuna, cod and salmon, since many types are contaminated with PCBs or mercury (or both). Select small oily fish, such as sprats and whitebait. Find safe, pure supplies or get your omega oils from cod liver oil (such as Carlson's or Nordic Naturals).

- Avoid artificial food additives of all kinds, especially artificial sweeteners such as aspartame, and non-organic foods, processed foods and those with added phosphates, artificial colouring, E numbers, artificial flavourings, sulphur agents and flavour enhancers such as MSG, and soy sauce.

- Wash all fruits and vegetables to remove pesticide residue.

- Avoid chemicals that have 'chloro' in their names, especially wood preservatives, herbicides and insecticides.

- Avoid chlorine bleach and any products that contain it. Substitutes are available, such as oxygen bleach.

- Don't buy or use products made of PVC (polyvinyl chloride); for example, clingfilm.

- Avoid using artificial air fresheners, fabric softeners and tumble-dryer fresheners. If you can smell it, there are molecules going up your nose!

- Have your tap water tested and, if contaminants are found, install an appropriate water filter such as a reverse osmosis filter. (Tap water contains chlorine, fluoride, solvents, pesticide residues and antibiotics.)

- Furnishing fabrics/mattresses, and so on, contain flame retardants such as PBDEs (polybrominated diphenyl ethers), chemical agents and fabric softeners. Try to buy furnishing fabrics and mattresses that have not been treated; you can get these through organic suppliers, such as Abaca Mattresses.

- Think carefully about vaccinations if your child is unwell at all. In my opinion vaccinations are very dangerous to those infants who may well be genetically predisposed with a dysfunctional immune system, or those who have problems dealing with additional toxins and heavy metals. I gave my youngest *no* vaccinations but appreciate that this is totally a parental decision.

- Avoid using indoor and outdoor chemicals. Read the labels, as most cleaning products are hazardous.

- Avoid perfumes, shampoos, conditioners, soaps, body lotions and fragrances that contain phthalates. Many individuals with an ASC find it difficult to detoxify and many are sensitive to certain fragrances, body lotions, soaps and shampoos, so these should be avoided by those individuals who are sensitive.

- Avoid plastics. These contain bisphenol A, phthalates, PFOA (perfluorooctanoic acid), formaldehyde, and PDBEs (polybrominated diphenyl ethers). Any chemical foreign to the body cannot be utilised and must therefore be excreted, and as a result will put pressure on an individual's health.

- Avoid non-stick saucepans and cookware, as these contain PFOA, linked with cancer and developmental problems.

- Avoid manufactured wood products, such as plywood and panelling, as well as glues and adhesives. These contain formaldehyde, causing cancer, nausea and skin irritations.

I recognise that this is a long list, but remember that chemicals cannot be utilised by the body. They therefore cause harm by disrupting many of our bodily functions, such as blocking certain enzymes. Furthermore, they are carcinogenic, and they reduce energy production by blocking the chemical pathways that make energy in each cell, and they therefore have to be excreted.

Recently, a child came into my clinic who was eating coloured sweets to the extent that his tongue was turquoise. I asked the mother if I could leave the room for a minute, and then returned with a purple board marker and asked if I could colour his tongue purple. She was horrified and said of course not, I then replied that I only wanted to do exactly the same thing that she was doing. Many parents are simply unaware of these toxins, as they have been consuming them since before they can remember; but now it is time to wake up and understand the serious effects of these unnatural products.

Drugs: a 'foreign' toxin

The reason why drugs have sometimes to be given continuously is because they are prescribed to address a symptom but not the cause. The body therefore removes them in the same way that it naturally gets rid of foreign, unwanted toxins. When the symptoms return, the drug is again administered to address the symptom.

As an example, if depression is diagnosed for an individual, a serotonin reuptake inhibiting drug (or SSRI) is prescribed to increase the levels of serotonin between the nerve cells; the symptoms of depression then decrease. The body removes the drug and the symptoms return. If the cause, which might be inflammation, is not addressed then depression will continue.

You will have seen from this chapter that toxic exposure is surrounding us; we are living in a toxic soup and consuming toxic products; we sleep on toxic mattresses, drink toxic water, eat toxic foods and, as a result, they are putting us all at risk. If you have been predisposed with an inability to remove toxins efficiently and effectively from your body, as would seem to be the case with many individuals with an ASC, it is time to adjust. By doing this you will not only support yourself but also your child, your other family members and anyone who enters your home.

In the next chapter Polly describes the effects that having a child with autism have on the whole family and suggests ways of coping with the diagnosis and with the reactions of others.

CHAPTER 6

Feelings and Family Life

As soon as the formal diagnosis came for Billy, so did the emotions. I had no idea how strong these would be. I didn't want anyone to talk to me and I didn't want to talk to anyone else about Billy until Jon and I had got our heads around this.

The phones rang; we didn't answer. This was our way of dealing with it. Other people will deal with it in different ways.

There is no single solution, as we all react in distinct ways. If there is any advice I can give you, it is to recognise that you have to work through your emotions, and allow yourself to be sad, to be angry, or whatever you are feeling, for as long as it takes.

I have said many times before that you are not on your own, as sadly there are too many who have been there before you and many who will come after. I am 'through it' now. I never thought I'd get there, but I have. There are still times when something will happen and I'll have the odd cry, but it is what it is, and crying actually does sometimes make you feel a lot better afterwards.

From the experience of my own journey, I know that despite the initial feeling of devastation, you will get through it, even though at the time of diagnosis it feels as if the bottom has dropped out of your world and that things couldn't get any worse. Times have changed since Billy was diagnosed; there is now more help and support than ever, although there is still not enough. There are many brilliant and determined parents and professionals out there who are fighting for change and better support for our children. When you have the strength, you may even decide to join them. Nothing helps the healing process better than throwing yourself into something positive that you know will benefit your child and their future.

In this chapter I am going to share some of our experiences from our own emotional journey, and some examples of the many calls and emails I have had on the subject of how different people have dealt with the often devastating diagnosis of autism in their child. I hope that by setting out a few of the totally normal and understandable emotions, you may recognise similarities. Hopefully, something here may just help.

The pain of loss

The most common feeling that so many parents talk about is a huge feeling of loss. Most talk about the loss of 'the child they thought they were having', what they thought their lives and that of their child would have been; others talk about the loss of the child they say they had before.

One mother wrote, 'The pain is immense. I ache for the little boy I thought he would be. I ache for my son, hoping that his new life will be a safe one where no one will hurt him. We live in a cruel world. The sympathy from others doesn't help.'

Another mother said, 'It's not like he is dead or anything, but right now I feel he might as well be; this is not the son I gave birth to.' This mother was deeply sad but also angry – another common emotion. I know her well, however, and she has also 'come through', as I did, and now runs a support group helping others.

I firmly believe that you must never feel guilty about how you feel; it is to be expected and completely natural that you will go through a number of emotions that you have never experienced to this degree before.

It really is a horribly complex set of emotions, partly because, as a loving parent, you don't want to seem to be 'disappointed' with your child, and want to feel that you wouldn't want him or her any other way, but you perhaps actually feel that the hopes and dreams you had about having this child have been crushed. Your child's life and your life will not be what you hoped they would be. This is not what you 'signed up for' and you have been robbed of the family you wanted.

Perhaps the loss you feel is the loss of what you thought your role and relationship as a parent would be. You've been denied your vision of motherhood or fatherhood and have been dealt something else instead.

As if it wasn't painful enough, you may also hate yourself for feeling this way. Whatever it is, however you feel cannot be wrong, if it's truly how you feel, although other people will struggle to understand, unless they've been through it or are going through it themselves. Unless you can talk about it with people you trust, you will have to cope with the grief, the anger, the disappointment, the resentment, the fear, the sadness, or whatever you're feeling, on your own, and you may have to excuse others for not automatically understanding what you're going through.

It could be, of course, that that's exactly how you cope best. Perhaps the last thing you want to do is open up your deepest emotions to friends or to sit in a room with strangers who may be coping with a similar situation in an entirely different way.

No one can tell you how you should be feeling, or how you should grieve or how you should see it (although some may try); but once you've found a way through the initial shock and have begun to figure out how you feel, sharing your thoughts and feelings can be an immensely helpful part of the process, whether this is with close friends or family, a support group or just your partner.

Some people find it helpful to think of this part of their complex emotions as a process akin to bereavement. It's not the same of course, as you still have your child, and your love for him or her, and the relationship you have and the support you will give are separate and distinct from this; but if you feel a sense of loss, you may find it helpful to acknowledge to yourself that you will need to live through unpredictable stages of grief for the child and the life you thought you had.

For others, this is not a helpful or meaningful approach. After all, no one knows in advance what their child will be like, and what's important is dealing with the reality you're faced with. Nevertheless, you will still be deluged with a variety of strong emotions.

However you feel about it, it is important to accept that everyone has their own way, and no one's way is wrong, and if you discuss it with no one else, do discuss it with your partner, and be prepared to accept that he or she may be experiencing a different set of emotions and may need to cope in an entirely different way from you. It is terribly sad but true that relationships can be put under a dreadful strain by having a child with autism, or indeed any disability or special need, and much of this strain can arise from differences in the way each person in the relationship feels and copes, particularly if these emotions remain unspoken or suppressed.

The most difficult thing to see right now is that you will get through it, that you won't always feel these emotions so overwhelmingly fiercely, that your life may be different from what you thought you'd planned, but will be every bit as full of joy and love and pride and fun and heartache.

First feelings

If you're a parent:
- As someone who has experienced this, I can say that you *will* get through.
- OK, this is not what you had mapped out for your child, but it's a different journey and there are many people out there who can help you.
- Allow yourself to go through this emotion. It's all right and it will make you stronger.

- If you can, talk to your partner. You are going through this together.

If you want to help a parent:

- Be there for them but don't offer 'it will be OK' words – they don't help.

- Look for local support groups; write down a list of people who may be able to help. Don't do any more than just hand the list to them. Words don't help at this point; they need time.

- Make sure they know you are there if they need you.

Your feeling of fear

Another feeling you may have is fear. Fear that your child is going to wreck the family; fear that you are not going to be able to help him or her; fear that you won't cope or won't have the strength. Fear of the unknown.

Suddenly, you find yourselves faced with a whole bunch of unknowns and variables that no one has ever prepared you for. You have no frame of reference for the parenting skills, coping strategies and sheer logistics of the task that lies before you – and it's terrifying. What if you can't do it? What if you try and fail? What if you make the wrong decisions or can't agree on which is the right one? You know other people cope, so if you can't cope, how will this reflect on you, your commitment, your dedication and your value as a parent?

What will happen to your child and to your family? What will his life be like? What will your life be like? You will ask, 'Am I strong enough?', 'Are we strong enough?'

Some time ago I spoke to a father who rang me to say he couldn't cope any more and didn't want to ever go home. He was frightened, frightened of his marriage going down the tubes because he and his wife were both so tired – they constantly shouted at each other and blamed each other. He felt completely alone and unsupported, he had hit rock bottom and he wanted to end his life. He was in a state of fear and panic, and it was the fear and panic talking. Actually, what he needed was someone to talk to; someone to whom he could articulate his fears and his anger and bitterness without the blame he felt had built up between him and his wife. Over time I got to know this man and he's now fine. He went back home that night and told his wife how he was feeling; he cried with her, they got some family help and are both now active campaigners for better support for families with autism.

It is vital that in trying to cope you have someone you can talk to. Unfortunately, I know that that is easier said than done. I remember someone saying that to me: 'Talk to someone apart from Jon. He can't help you, because he's suffering too.' The trouble I found was that no one else understood. How could they? The only people who could begin to understand were other families living with autism and my husband, Jon – people who could empathise, not just sympathise.

Of course, there are many people who might be able to help, including support groups and helplines set up for exactly this purpose, and people who specialise in helping with complex emotions like these for individuals and for families. Often the difficulty is in recognising that you need help or acknowledging that someone who's not going through what you're going through could possibly understand enough to offer the support you need.

When Billy was aged two, we had just been on the *Tonight with Trevor McDonald* programme. We were taking a well-earned break on Tresco, a small island in the Scillies (my late father worked there, so we were lucky to have regular holidays in this beautiful place). The island is tiny with a very close community and everyone knows each other. Also on the island were many visitors, most of whom we also knew well. One of my father's friends was visiting that week, a good family friend. The day after the TV show was broadcast I was walking down the winding Tresco roads with Dad, when suddenly this friend came up to me and said, 'I saw you, Billy and your family on the television last night. Let me give you some advice. There are many good residential schools that will take Billy; you really must send him away. There are people that will support Billy, then you and your family can get on with your life. He's a sweet boy but I've seen this before, it breaks a family up.' I politely thanked him, walked along a few more roads with Dad with neither of us saying anything. Eventually I said, 'Dad, I could never send Billy away. I don't know how we are going to get through this, but he stays with us.' It was that friend of my father's fear for the rest of the family that made him come to what he felt was the best solution for my family. I'm very glad I didn't take that advice.

Here are some suggestions that I hope might help you:

- Don't be frightened – you are not on your own.
- Fear is usually based on 'the unknown' or feelings of powerlessness to stop something bad from happening. Read as much as you can on autism to turn 'the unknown' into 'the known' and to give yourself the power to affect change. Use our recommended reading list in Resources to guide you.
- Remember, you are this child's parents; you will have the strength to do this. It will have its tough times, but also there will be extraordinary times that will make your life more blessed than most.

Coping with guilt

Guilt is another emotion that most parents feel. For Jon and me, our guilt was because we felt that we could have prevented Billy's autism. Billy was so 'normal', so 'typical' in his first year, and then everything changed because of a decision we made. I still wonder to this day how Billy would be if I hadn't given him the MMR vaccination, or maybe if I had waited a year for his immune system to build up. That guilt will never leave me, and nothing and no one will ever be able to make it go away. Ultimately I am Billy's mother, my job was, and continues to be, to protect him until he can fend for himself. I didn't follow my instincts and I allowed a cocktail of powerful drugs and vaccinations to damage him.

Guilt is tough to deal with because, regardless of what any-one tells you, only you can deal with your own feelings of guilt. I've had endless disagreements with people who say to me, 'You mustn't feel guilty.' I do know that. It makes perfect sense in theory, but it makes no difference in reality because I still do. My way of easing the guilt is to throw myself into everything I can to make Billy's life better. Jon is the same. We don't talk about it or cry about it anymore, we just get on with it. So, as an advance warning to those of you who may write and try to tell me differently: it's my guilt and I'm dealing with it in the best way I know how.

Paul Shattock OBE has a son with autism. He is director of the Autism Research Unit at the University of Sunderland and founding chairman of European Services for People with Autism (ESPA). If you don't know Paul then you must Google him, contact him, know about him – he is a genius and is known to us in the UK as 'the godfather of autism'! Paul is a great source of information and a huge support to me and many others. He tells me that 'guilt is a terrible emotion, but one we all live with'.

Guilt is essentially a healthy emotion. It's there to help you to address the things you think you've done wrong so that you don't repeat those mistakes in the future. Unfortunately, feelings of guilt still arise even if you haven't done anything wrong, but feel somehow that 'things would be different if ...' Clearly, you can't change the past, but you can take steps to deal with your feelings of guilt in the present and future. For some people, the only way to do this is to do your utmost to 'make amends' or to find a way to lessen the impact of whatever it is you feel you've done wrong.

If you are suffering from guilt, throw yourself into something that will enhance your child's life. Maybe help a charity or a support group. It works for me. Write your feelings down, I get many articles sent to me for the *Autism File* about this – it can make you feel so much better. Other suggestions are:

- Use this emotion to do something positive for your child – anything that keeps you busy and has a satisfying end.

- Talking to people is very valuable. It may help you to see things differently, and just airing it can help you feel better about yourself. Talk to anyone who makes you feel better. If they understand, great, if not, move on.

- Remember, if people haven't lived through this, they simply won't understand how you are feeling. Don't get cross with them, do something different with them.

- If you find yourself feeling guilty that you're not doing enough to help your child, then you only really have two options: either remind yourself that you're doing all you can under the circumstances, or do more.

The moments of embarrassment

I would like to say to you, 'Never, ever feel embarrassed about your child.' This is obviously the right sentiment and a nice one; however, the trouble is that it doesn't always work like that.

When Billy was around five years old, we had used lots of bio-medical intervention with him, he was starting speech therapy and he was even saying a few words, so I felt we were ready to attempt a visit to our friends in Hampshire. They were good friends, so I had no worries. After a few hours with them, Jon and I said how wonderful this time was: all the children were playing happily together (Billy was at least in the same room – so that was good enough for us); the sun was out and we were actually having the first normal few hours in over four years. I will never forget what happened next. My friend came out into the garden and casually said, 'Is Billy thirsty – because he's drinking the water from our loo?' I looked at Jon; he looked at me. End of normality. My first feeling was of complete embarrassment. I couldn't help it. The only thing that I know drinks water from loos is a dog. Not my five-year-old son. Then anger: what was Billy doing? I had spent months teaching him to drink from a cup – he knows what to do. More anger and then resentment towards my friend: why did she have to come out and say that? Of course, Billy must be bloody thirsty, why else would he be drinking from the loo? Why didn't she stop him, give him a cup of water and never mention it?

Our blissful sense of wonderful normality was transformed in an instant to the draining, aching feeling that autism had brought to our lives.

So we left, and drove back in silence, the mood destroyed and the fun over. Again the siblings lost out, as they so often did.

Embarrassment is a tricky one to define and, at the time, there's absolutely nothing you can do about it. It's an automatic response caused by your perception of the 'transgression of social norms' and is actually a feature of a strong sense of social empathy: sharing the thoughts and feelings of others. People who don't understand or care about the perceptions of others don't tend to get embarrassed.

As such, feelings of embarrassment about the behaviour of your child are an unwanted acknowledgement to yourself of how other people might judge you and your child if they don't automatically understand all the complex reasons for this behaviour – which most people don't.

The better you know people and, more importantly, the more they know about your child and autism and how it affects your daily lives, the less likely you are to be embarrassed by 'unexpected' behaviour in front of them. A few strategies:

- If you feel embarrassed by people's responses to your child's behaviour when out in public, sometimes just saying 'he has autism' is enough to prompt people's ignorance into understanding. Otherwise, just remind yourself that it's their ignorance at fault, not you or your child. (See 'Cultivating understanding' on page 117.)

- Things that happen that seem like the end of the world at the time never are, and you really will laugh one day.

- Never build yourself up for a disappointment. When Billy first waved goodbye, I raced around to a friend's house to show her Billy's new skill. She just looked at me sadly when he wouldn't/couldn't do it. Moral of the story: don't expect too much from your child too quickly.

- Your child's skills and overall development can never be taken for granted in a new situation, so be prepared. Don't expect your child to learn too quickly or be able to do something in one place just because he has learned to in another.

When resentment arises

Resentment is a big one; a deep emotion that so many people don't admit to. We can't, because if we do then in the eyes of the world we become a really awful and bitter human being. But when you are extremely low, it can happen to anyone.

When Billy was at his worst, with his head-banging, his high-pitched screams and his tantrums if we tried to go anywhere or stop his precious *Spot the Dog* videos, a friend came round with her son who was a little younger than Billy. She complained from the minute she walked through my door about how her son had taken ages to be potty trained, 'He's a lazy nightmare!', she said. She moaned about how other children his age were doing multiplication in double numbers, 'But not my lazy little one.' She told me how he had been 'a joke' at the school sports day, but, 'Hey ho, we are all going to the cinema tonight to get over it.' (Cinema? I would give my right arm to be able to sit in a cinema with my family, let alone potty train, attend sports day and deal with multiplication with Billy.)

When she had left, I made a mental note to drop this friend completely. How dare she come into my house with her child doing things that I would give my life for and tell me he was lazy? I immediately resented her and I also resented her child. Shocking, I know, but for a very short moment those feelings were real. Thankfully, it was a short-lived emotion; poor Jon had to endure a night of me ranting on about this, but the next day I had moved on.

I deal with it differently now. When people say things like, 'Oh, my son only got 60 per cent in English', I change the subject (mainly because it seriously bores me) or ignore it. Occasionally, still, the resentment overflows and I might say 'Well, you're talking to a mum with a child who, when faced with a SATs test, couldn't even sit down on his chair, let alone understand the first question', then I smile and change the subject, knowing that this will undoubtedly make them feel uncomfortable. Childish? Yes, but fantastically rewarding on occasions.

Of course you will come across people who simply won't understand that what they're saying, or what their child's doing, may be a stark reminder of what your child can't do, and brings those feelings of loss and guilt and anger to the surface. Of course, they're entitled to their own perceptions and disappointments about their own child, but sometimes the resentment is simply unavoidable.

Resentment will ease, but it will still very occasionally hit you, so expect it. It'll be strongest when you are struggling to get your head around what you can do for your child, but try not to get too bogged down with it. It won't help you or your child.

Your true friends will know you well, and will be sensitive to your feelings, whether rational or not, and the more you talk to them the more they'll understand. I found that I simply decided not to see too much of people who said these things without thinking, and made new friends in the autism world who automatically understood and could empathise. There are unfortunately enough of us! Your old friends will stick with you if they were true friends in the first place. Autism has a way of sorting real friends from fair-weather friends, and Jon and I have lost people we thought were close friends – godparents to our children – through serious disagreements on autism. I remind myself often that these people could not have been who I thought they were.

I have had so many calls and emails from parents when they first get the diagnosis of autism saying, 'Why me? What have I done to deserve this? Why my child? Why isn't it someone who eats badly, smokes, drinks … Why me?' The unfairness is tough to take, but you have to avoid the slippery slope of blame seeking; it doesn't go anywhere.

Of course, the question remains: why us? We simply don't know. The jury is out, but many doctors and scientists are working around the world to find the answers, and we have to rely on them to work it out.

Meanwhile, we have to get over our hand wringing and blame game as parents. We have children with autism – that's the way it is, and they need our help.

I wasted too long crying, blaming and shouting. It's a waste of time and valuable energy that should be spent on our children – on Billy and his brother and sister.

A few suggestions:

- Try not to dwell on the 'Why me?' The bottom line is that it *is* us, we are strong and we are going to deal with this.

- It may seem harsh, but having a child with autism will help to clarify who your real friends are. If you can, let them know how you feel, and don't see friends who bring you down. They'll either get the idea, or they weren't true friends to begin with.

- So much is known about autism now. There is an answer for almost every problem you have. Bury your head in looking for those answers rather than dwelling on the past and what might have been.

Finding you are lonely

Loneliness is a painfully common emotion for families dealing with autism. It can seem as if the diagnosis has instantly isolated you from the rest of the world and that you have to cope alone with a new and frightening reality while everyone else carries on around you with the old familiar one that you no longer have access to.

Many feel lonely mainly because they simply can't do the things other families do.

I tried to take Billy to a playgroup with Bella and Toby, but we were asked to leave within half an hour as Billy was banging their kitchen door over and over again while I was running around after a crawling Toby. I was asked to find a more 'suitable' play-group. That was then, over ten years ago. Now there are many more special groups and places where we can take our little ones and their brothers and sisters. And if you live in an area where there is nothing, then gather some other mums and dads together and start one up.

One mother rang me to say how desperate she felt, like a prisoner in her own home. Her husband was never there and couldn't cope. The few times he did come home he was exhausted and went to bed. She had no family nearby, she didn't see friends any more and she felt she had no life beyond looking after her child who couldn't speak, ask for anything or show any interest in any toys. This mother was lonely and isolated. As it happened, we had a few readers of the *Autism File* in her area, I called them and they were more than happy to step in. They now have a support group together. The point really is that if you are in a situation as desperate as this mother you must do something about it. With the stats as high as they are in this country, you can guarantee another mother or father of autism with be close by.

You'll meet the best friends ever in the autism world. Today there is no need to be lonely, as there are so many of us. Autism mothers and fathers are everywhere.

- If you feel isolated because you feel the people around you –
  your friends, family or even your partner – don't understand
  what you're going through, or don't realise that you need help
  and support, tell them. It's fine to need help and support. We
  all need it.

- Find the right playgroup/support group. Very few areas these
  days don't have one. Your doctor, health visitor, social worker
  or school should be able to help. Try typing 'autism support
  group' and your town into a search engine.

- Even if you aren't 'a joiner' you'll find help and support, and a
  ready-made community in online groups and forums. See our
  recommended sites at the end of this book.

- Look for like-minded families living with autism, they will
  help and be valuable friends. As soon as you get involved in a
  support group, or start a home programme, or take up a
  school or nursery place, you will find people who share your
  experience.

- Remember, if the stats are 1 in 100, there will be a family going
  through exactly what you are very close to you.

Cultivating understanding

There are many situations that I have encountered where a
simple lack of understanding causes unpleasant scenes. It's difficult to advise on how to cope every time, but by sharing it may
just help!

One of many examples with Billy was about shoes. From the
age of two until he was about nine Billy hated having new shoes
and we dreaded taking him, but we had a good relationship with
a local shoe shop and they knew the deal. We would pick what we
hoped was a quiet time (we'd ring them in advance) and I would
take Billy along with support in tow.

On this occasion Bella and I 'braved it'. As usual, Billy threw
himself on the floor screaming his head off as soon as I removed

his shoes. So I sat on Billy (gently, but firmly) while the sales assistant attempted to put the new ones on in between trying not to get kicked. Eventually the task was done, fairly quickly but extremely stressfully. Billy then carried on screaming while I paid, and I was expecting to get him to the car, after which the whole incident would be forgotten. On this occasion though, while I was paying, I was suddenly aware of a middle-aged woman shouting at Billy. Bella was standing rooted to the spot, crying. 'I feel sorry for your parents having a rude child like you. You are an utter disgrace, a spoilt, horrid little monster', yelled the woman at Billy.

The thing was that Bella was the one that suffered. Billy didn't hear or care, he just carried on screaming. He didn't even know the woman was shouting at him. Bella, in contrast, was shaking with fear. I walked straight up to Bella, took her hand, pulled Billy up, ignored the awful woman and headed out. Once in the safety of the car, I comforted Bella. I didn't shout back or speak to the woman at the time as it would have made it even worse for Bella. Our lovely shoe shop rang later to say that they had explained to the woman that Billy had autism and the woman was extremely sorry. On hearing that, I told Bella. It's vitally important that when a sibling is affected by a situation they hear the conclusion, so that they can make sense of it. Otherwise it stays in their minds and they make their own conclusions up. Incidentally, as I write, Bella (who is now 15) tells me she has no memory of this!

I would like to think that the woman in question would think twice before acting that way again, and I hope the experience has taught her not to jump to conclusions or to interfere in an obviously difficult situation without any understanding of the circumstances.

It doesn't occur to most people that your child has autism and so is unable to cope with seemingly ordinary situations due to issues of physical sensitivity or changes in routine, and so on. It's simply out of most people's experience, and their first response is to assume that you have a naughty child, a spoilt child. In some twisted and ignorant way, that woman probably thought she was doing some good. It's easy in hindsight to put such incidents down to people's ignorance, but at the time it can be devastating.

We've still got a long way to go in educating the general public about the reality of autism, but most people know that there is a thing called autism, and that it will affect a child's behaviour. Clearly, if people weren't ignorant, then they wouldn't jump to conclusions, but that's not the way the world works – they are and they do.

Although it may seem difficult to swallow, and may be the last thing you want to do when faced with ignorance and assumption, we who know need to take some responsibility for informing people about autism. Sometimes, the simple explanation 'my son has autism' can diffuse an otherwise difficult situation, may lead to wider understanding, and may even bring offers of support rather than judgement and condemnation.

- Some people find it helpful to carry cards or leaflets with them that explain autism, and may help to rationalise your child's behaviour and the plight of all people with autism to people who would otherwise remain ignorant. You don't have to engage with them, just give them a card.

- The more you understand about your child's particular sensitivities and needs, the more you will be able to prepare yourself for situations that you know are going to be difficult.

- If you see children 'behaving badly', don't jump to conclusions. Why not assume that, for whatever reason, this is a difficult time for the child and for the parents (and siblings).

- Spread the word. People may understand that your child has autism, but do they understand what this means? The more you know about the underlying causes of your child's different and wonderful behaviours, the better equipped you will be to explain them. The more people know, the better the future will be for our children!

The effects of bullying

Bullying is a major issue, linked to a lack of understanding. Children with autism are different. Some may be intellectually bright, but even those who are academically able are bound to be socially naive and gauche; they wouldn't be autistic if they weren't. Unfortunately, this difference can lead to bullying by people who don't know better and are acting on their own, ignorant agenda. This is one of the many reasons why mainstream school might not be right for a child with an ASC, however bright they are. It is a hard pill to swallow that intellectual capability or academic prowess is not what it takes to survive and thrive in school or command respect in the community. For those children who are clearly different and not academically gifted, it can be even worse. The reality is that the social difficulties faced by our children are far more significant and far more important than any academic achievement, as it is social and vocational skills, not academic skills that lead to a happy and fulfilled life.

Many children with autism are subjected to bullying, but I also speak to many parents who tell me that the brothers and sisters of our children with autism are also prone to bullying, particularly in school.

We first encountered this when Bella was seven years old. Bella came home one day with a serious face. 'Mummy,' she said, 'no one in my class apart from Sophie wants to come home to play. They say that they don't want to catch Billy's disease.' I looked down at my little girl as she fought hard to hold back the tears welling in her big eyes. I sat her down and calmly told her that the children in the class just needed to be shown what autism is and understand that you certainly can't catch it! Inside I was furious, furious with the other children, furious with their parents who obviously knew no better, and pretty livid with the school.

The next morning I marched into the school and demanded to see both the Head and Bella's class teacher. In fact the school was horrified by the revelation, and turned out to be brilliant at dealing with it. Bella's teacher took her aside and together they hatched a plan. So that day she came bouncing out of school, 'Guess what Mummy, we had circle time and my teacher talked about a little boy who had autism. She told us that he was different but learning in another way that's easier for him and that people have to be very patient and help him understand. Then she asked if anyone knew anyone with autism but before I could put my hand up Sarah said her cousin had it, and then I talked about Billy. Now we have to all write poems about special people.'

I have to say I was touched by the poem Bella wrote.

My Brother Billy by Bella Tommey, age seven

What's going to happen to my brother Billy?
The boy who everyone thinks is so silly,
Is he going to relish the wonder we will?
Nobody knows what the future will spill.

Most people think he won't be that clever,
But actually he will be, forever and ever,
His talents are greater than you can imagine,
A top one is that magnificent grin.

He is kind and benevolent,
So if there ever occurs an accident,
Billy will always be there on the scene,
Wiping the wounds so you are fresh and clean.

My brother Billy thinks he's a dog,
He barks and asks you to throw him a log,
He asks to sit in the boot of our car,
But Mummy says that's going too far.

Billy is also a rally car king,
He wins and wins until finally he sings,
His joy echoing through the house,
Until everyone in the family is up in a rouse!

My brother Billy has autism, you know,
And I'm not really sure when it's going to go,
Even when it's time to call it quits,
I'll obviously still love him to bits.

What's going to happen to my brother Billy?
The boy who everyone thinks is so silly,
Some people say he is bad or mad,
But that just makes our family sad.

So, be kind to my brother called Billy.

I spoke to one mother who rang in a panic to tell me that her nine-year-old had got into a fight at his school because another boy had said his brother with autism was a 'freak'. The mother, who secretly said to me (of course, not to the boy in question) how proud she was of her son, wrote letters to all the parents in the school explaining about autism and how tough it was for her other son to cope with it. She then asked the parents to explain to their children about autism to make things easier for her son. It worked.

People need to be told, as it is general ignorance and lack of understanding that causes these problems and I am a real believer that education, training and support are the key here.

Bella's and Toby's friends love Billy and often take time out to be on the Play Station or computer with him. So, my simple advice here is to tell everyone about autism, as once people understand, the majority are fantastically helpful.

Children can be terribly cruel to each other. They are search-ing for meaning and acceptance; they are learning how to 'be' within a group and seeking their place in the hierarchy of their peers. Sometimes this involves asserting their own place and rejecting anything or anyone that is different, or who 'sticks out' from their own understanding of the social norm, if only to show their peers that they 'understand' and that they are worthy to remain part of the group. Unfortunately, this translates as per-secution of the weak or different by the strong and dominant, and it overflows into persecution of anyone associated with the weak or different in the jostling for social position.

Anyone who is different from the crowd is vulnerable to bully-ing, and even those who aren't essentially different, but are weaker, will be affected by the unpleasantness of social rejection.

This is a fact of life, and is entirely normal within any society, but it is entirely unfair to people who aren't able to compete socially, or who have this association through no fault of their own. Bella's story shows that much of this is down to ignorance (again) and that, furnished with the right information, it is possi-ble to shift the accent in a group from ignorance and bullying to knowledge, acceptance and even protection.

Of course, there are many children (and adults) out there who will happily take the perceived kudos or self-gratification from dominating any other person, without ever stopping (or having the ability) to think about what they are doing, but there really is little we can do about these people, and everyone comes across them at some point in their lives. Some ideas for ways to deal with bullying are:

- Move in as soon as you feel a sibling or your child with autism has been/is being bullied.
- Remember, generally people just don't understand, they need to be told/shown.
- All schools will have a policy for dealing with this sort of thing.

Using support groups

Support groups matter. There are, of course, good ones and not so good ones, depending on your own personality and point of view. When I had just got Billy's diagnosis, I found a little support group in our area. I didn't want to go initially because I suppose it confirmed to me that I was an 'Autism Mother', something I am very proud to be now. But I went along, mainly hoping that someone could give me some direction, some idea of what on earth to do about it.

Learning how to control Billy would be good I thought, as Billy was a living nightmare at this stage and no one I met anywhere seemed to know how to help him or even what autism was. So off I went. A lady answered the door and kindly offered me a cup of tea and a biscuit. I immediately felt uncomfortable. Some readers might have liked this group, but for me and the way I am I knew straight away that it wasn't going to be my thing. One by one, others started to arrive, and about 12 parents came. Everyone sat around chatting, but it was all very quiet – it reminded me of a wake.

My character is such that, if there's a problem, my response will be, 'Let's talk about it and find an answer or a solution.' These quiet ladies were different. They talked about their shopping, about the book clubs they had joined, about a new dish available in Sainsbury's. After half an hour I had had enough. I (possibly slightly aggressively) asked in a very loud voice if someone could actually give me some advice about my son. I explained that Billy would only turn right outside our front door, when nine times out of ten I really needed to turn left, as right went nowhere for a very long time. If you tried to encourage Billy to turn left he went absolutely berserk, only Jon had managed it on a few occasions, but Billy had screamed for hours. The conversation went something like this:

Lady 1: 'Difficult … my daughter has never done that.'

Lady 2: (followed by the rest): 'Nor mine … no, never.'

So now I was thinking that Billy must be so much worse than anyone else's child – maybe there was something else wrong with him?

Lady 1: 'Have you tried your health visitor?'

That was enough for me – try my health visitor? My health visitor barely knew what autism was. I politely (although maybe not, as I seem to remember being slightly rude – another example of trying to cope) left after this exchange, vowing never to go to a support group again.

The point of this story is that this particular group simply wasn't for me and the kind of person I am. There was nothing wrong with the group, as the other 12 members obviously found comfort and support in calmly talking about everyday things. I can now see how comforting it may be to be able to talk about the mundanities of life with people who understand how extraordinary these may be, but this was not what I needed at the time. I did, however, find other groups subsequently that helped enormously, and people who were able to share similar experiences and empathise with mine. They helped me feel less isolated, less different, less resentful, and guided me towards further help and support. If there's a moral to this story, it is that we are all different, and that, as is the case in life in general, shared experience isn't necessarily an indicator of shared values.

Just be careful that you don't get 'brainwashed' by well-meaning parents that tell you that you *have* to follow their journey, what worked for them. Take what you need from their experiences and then look at your child – and remember that you know your child the best.

An example of this involved Billy when he was around three years old. Billy was very noise sensitive and his sister Bella was given a keyboard for her birthday. If she even played one note on it, he would run over and bite, kick or hit her – anything to stop her playing. Billy would cover his ears and scream. There were many other examples that showed us that Billy was struggling with noise. Therefore, at a support group meeting (yes, I did try another one!) I asked an experienced mother (the one who everyone went to with all their problems, as generally she really helped us) what I should do and whether she had heard of a therapy called AIT (auditory integration therapy). This is what she said:

Autism Mother: 'Yes, I have, but it's rubbish. I tried it on my son – it was a waste of money.'

Me: 'Where did you go? Did your son have the same problems as Billy?'

Autism Mother: 'I can't remember, but they're all the same. Don't even bother. It won't work and it's expensive.'

After a week or so of Billy beating us all up every time we turned the radio on or even listened to any music, I had had enough. I called the AIT place and booked Billy in. It was one of the best things I have ever done. In no time Billy's noise sensitivity was history. So, again, you are in charge – he or she is your child. That well-meaning and experienced mother was adamant about AIT, because she didn't want me to waste my time and money because her experiences had been bad. Great advice, but wrong for Billy. When I advise other parents now, I tend to say, 'It did/didn't work for Billy, but others have said it has/hasn't for them.'

Marriage: staying together

Tricky one this, as according to a study by the National Autism Association, 85 per cent of marriages that involve a child with autism will end. There is no doubt that autism puts a strain on a relationship. It's hardly surprising; first of all we are exhausted, and many of us have little money because we have thrown everything we have at autism. If Jon and I row it's always because we are tired and overworked. The most important thing that Jon and I do is have some time together every evening to talk. Admittedly this is over a glass of wine, generally, but it gives us a chance to go over our days and bounce ideas off each other. Someone told me once about autism and relationships: if your relationship is weak, it will become weaker; if it is strong it becomes stronger. Autism will exaggerate every aspect of your marriage. That said, there are times when you will question whether you have a strong marriage, it will be inevitable, when you are overtired you question everything. Writing about how to keep a relationship strong when you are dealing with autism is difficult because keeping a strong relationship without autism can be hard enough. Here are some tips that some might say are easier said than done, but nonetheless are ones that have worked for many of us that are still together. One piece of advice a well-meaning friend gave me once made me really think, and I did make a concerted effort; it's blunt but it certainly gave me a wake-up call. She said, 'Always remember there is another woman waiting to pounce, if you don't look after your husband, then another one will.' This works both ways. Sometimes our lives are so consumed with autism that it's easy to forget each other. The effort has to be put in or, like my friend said, someone else will. That said, I believe that if a marriage doesn't make it, then you must never feel guilty, it's incredibly hard, as the statistics show, to make everything work; we can only do our best.

- Find time to talk, even if it means getting a family member or friend round to give you half an hour or so together. Don't bottle up emotions; tell each other how you feel.

- Remember that your marriage needs attention, as well as your children.

- Even if it's time together flopping in front of the television, it's time out – we all need that.

- Physical contact is so important, even if it's just small.

- Tell each other how grateful you are for the things you both do – never take each other for granted.

- Focus on each other's positives rather than the negatives.
- Laugh whenever you can – even if you have to hire a comedy DVD!
- Try to give each other their own space. Look for a local yoga/Pilates class that will help you relax.

The effects on siblings

Siblings have a tough time when they have a brother or sister with autism. For Bella, being 16 months older than Billy, autism came into her little life when she was around three years old. Before autism hit us, in my quest to be the 'perfect mother', I would spend hours painting, cooking, reading and playing with my little girl. Billy would either be attached to my hip or happily crawling as he followed us around.

Billy's decline happened so quickly that Bella's life suddenly took a drastic turn, and on top of that I was pregnant with Toby. My attention was now solely focused on why Billy was sick with tummy problems, why he had dark eye circles, why his hair was falling out. Jon and I were both exhausted, and so Bella asking for any attention was now too much. My friend Heidi was a great source of help at this time. She would march round, scoop Bella up and take her for wonderful days out. Bella loved this, but for me it was a heady mixture of sadness and gratitude. I wanted to be the one to take Bella out, but that wasn't an option anymore. Billy needed my help and I was his mother.

I think I would do this differently if I had that time again. I was completely obsessive about being Billy's carer. I felt that only I could manage him. My advice to parents in the same situation today is to take a step back for a minute and think. It is hard when you are exhausted and emotional, but it is essential.

First of all, it clearly helps if you have the money to afford 'help'. I didn't and most don't, and I probably wouldn't have taken outside help on unless it was expert autism help; however, if you do have the money and you can afford it, I recommend that you find someone to help you by looking after your child for a minimum of an hour a day. If you can't, then find some good friends or members of the family to rotate and help out. It is important that you make it clear to the friends or family members helping out that you simply need time with your other children and that you don't need a running commentary on how shocked they are that your son/daughter with autism did this or that while in their charge. We know what our child does, we live with it 24/7. So unless our little autism cherubs do anything positive, we don't want to hear about it, thank you very much! So when they arrive, smile sweetly and get out fast! It's not that we're rejecting them; it's only that we need some time with the others – or even time just to be ourselves.

If I had been given an hour a day as a break from Billy, I would naturally have preferred to have slept, to have caught up on the never-ending housework, to have watched a mind-numbing soap, read a book – anything. The childhood years go so fast. Yes, you are tired, but please take my advice, and don't miss what you can get of your other children's childhood.

Without any doubt, I missed too much. I feel sad, especially for Toby, who is two years younger than Billy. By the time he was born, Jon and I were in full swing with the biomedical and therapy side for Billy. I hate to admit that I have only sketchy memories of Toby in his first year.

I recently watched a video of Toby at about five months old in one of those bouncy chairs. I used to put him in it and plonk him in any room where people were, so that he could at least interact. This video was sad. My little Toby was sitting in his chair looking around and if anyone walked by he would look up, kick his little legs and smile, desperate for someone's attention.

Today, both Bella and Toby are great children. They are both kind and will help anyone who has special needs of any kind. They empathise, understand and know 'the deal'. These days, sibling clubs are being set up either on the Internet or as groups, as it is fast becoming an essential realisation that autism affects the whole family. You will rarely see a more compassionate person than the sibling of a person with autism.

Family life

Because stress levels in our house were abnormally high, lack of sleep was a huge problem for all of us. In the early days, Billy would bang his head all night, literally getting just a couple of hours of sleep.

I would hear the dull thud of his head being walloped against the wall followed by crying. I used to lie in my bed until I could no longer stay awake, in despair, asking myself, 'Why?' What could we do to stop him doing this? It affected us all incessantly.

Doctors, people with autism and other 'experts' told us that the head-banging was a common trait of autism, they said it was 'frustration'. After so long and so many people telling you this was the case, you start to accept and believe it. We now know this simply wasn't the case. Once Jon started the biomedical treatments for Billy his head-banging stopped – so there was definitely something driving it.

As soon as we had conquered the head-banging, Billy moved on to singing all night! I agree this was much better than head-banging but it was still incredibly hard to get to sleep, as his volume levels changed dramatically.

The other children were tired, we were tired and it meant we snapped at each other. My advice to parents with this problem is that you mustn't let it go on for as long as we did. There are many things you can do to help your child sleep. A mixture of diet, bio-medical advice and getting good educational input is top of my list here. Different things work for different families. For us, it was through correcting Billy's health, his diet and by having a firmer hand. Billy got away with us saying, 'It's not his fault, he has autism', for too long. Even now with Billy at 14, we let him stay up later than we probably should, in the hope that we will get a reasonably late wake-up call from him. With Bella and Toby tired as well, it affected their everyday activities, and with us as snappy parents too they had a hard time.

As the children started to get older, Jon and I made a plan that we would spend a minimum of 20 minutes one-on-one with each child each day. It might not sound a lot, but if you don't put yourself under too much pressure then it's more likely to happen. So, Jon's favourite place to take Bella and Toby was to the local pub to chat with their dad over a glass of lemonade and a packet of crisps. They loved it and, of course, so did Jon! Other activities like sitting and doing a puzzle or playing a game with no interruptions helped as well, a trip to a café, cinema, anything that gives you quality time with that child. It makes a huge difference.

I have to say that the bond I see forming between all siblings of autism is unique. The love and strength they have for their brother or sister with autism is so powerful, unconditional and exceptional. The respect for each other, and others around the world as they join together through sibling groups, is also untold; the siblings are our children with autism's future.

It is without doubt a hard task being part of the extended family. Some say that the worst thing is when a member of the family (it tends to be the grandparents), won't accept that their grandchild has autism. Comments like, 'Oh, *you* were a late speaker', or 'Einstein didn't speak until he was six' really don't help. I have come to realise that this is the way that some people deal with it.

One grandmother said to me that it hurt so much to see her daughter suffer the pain with her son's diagnosis that she could barely bring herself to talk about autism. She would talk about anything else to try to keep her mind off something that she couldn't cope with.

People want to help, but many just don't know how to. Some try to 'take charge', but parents generally don't need or want that.

One mother once rang me in floods of tears saying that her

mother had all but moved in and was organising the daily routine of her child. Every time she tried to do something with her child her mother would say, 'Not like that. That's not right.'

I spoke to a grandmother recently who was desperate for some advice, as her daughter wasn't coping with her autistic son and refused to see anyone. She said her daughter seemed to be in denial and was depressed. What could she do?

It is complicated. Parents want help but not to be judged, but they really need help with the things that they don't have time for like ironing, cooking, shopping and cleaning.

If they need help with their child, they will ask for it.

My advice for a family wanting to help is:

- Accept the diagnosis.
- Talk to the family members dealing with autism and ask how you can help.
- Offer to do the everyday tasks or watch the children while they catch up on sleep or the rest of their lives.
- Don't take over and make unhelpful comments about the child with autism. Remember, the parents may be tired, oversensitive and still coming to terms with it.
- If you offer to take the children out, do include the child with autism; it's very hurtful when they are constantly left out.
- Talk to the parents about how their child is and whether you can help with any therapies or by developing new skills.
- Be there for them.

The extended family

Autism also affects members of the extended family. To illustrate this, I asked a few members of my own family to write a short piece about how they felt about Billy and the journey we have all been on.

My Grandson Has Autism

by Wendy Barber, Billy's Grandmother

The first time that I voiced my conviction that my grandson, Billy, had autism I was sitting in my doctor's surgery discussing routine matters and I heard myself say that Billy had autism. This was completely spontaneous, so what was I hoping to achieve? I think it was that in voicing this fear the professional would make it all go away. Of course, this does not happen and I doubt if the doctor had any more knowledge of autism than I did. Walking back, I was forced to face the reality. As far as I knew, my daughter and son-in-law had not had a formal diagnosis, but I was sure that they were worrying – both were avoiding discussing Billy's development with me. Near to tears and in despair for my daughter and her husband, I grappled with this new situation – new, because I had finally admitted to myself that it was time to accept that autism was now part of our lives. In fact it was to change the family forever.

Although I was mourning the loss of the 'typical' grandson we had welcomed 18 months earlier, my overriding sense of despair was for my lovely, lively daughter. All mothers will recognise the desire to take away pain from their children, if only we could. It is so hard to accept that your child is facing a traumatic situation; it is theirs and ultimately they must cope with it.

For years we had been a complacent family believing that these things didn't happen to us, we heard about other families with autism, it was remote, sad, but not our problem. Billy's diagnosis, when it did come, rocketed us all out of our comfort zone. My four newly wed children were all starting their families, and Polly was already expecting her third child. Now, every pregnancy had to be thought about in relation to the fact that autism was a possibility. Following the diagnosis, each of Billy's parental families looked back and analysed, 'Is it in my family?', 'Is it in your family?' 'Was so-and-so a bit odd?' The analysis begins of the parent's childhood, the environment, the immunisation pro-gramme, the feeding patterns, and so on. It would be so much easier for us all if we knew why: 'Why Polly's son?' my inner voice screams as the tears slide down my face.

As the grandmother, I can only offer Billy's parents and sib-lings support and love. Ultimately, the reality of the day-to-day pressures of bringing up a child with autism are dealt with by the parents; it's their responsibility, the sleepless nights, dealing with the fragile digestive disorders, lack of 'normal' develop-ment and explaining Billy's difference to strangers as his behaviour becomes noticeable. I stand by, helpless, aware that words of comfort are inadequate, not even helpful, and desper-ately wanting to take away the pain. I feel concern for Billy's siblings, as practically every decision the family makes has to take into account his autism. They cope well. But things are different, tougher.

All in all, Billy's diagnosis has not been the tragedy that we feared. Our beloved Billy, uniquely himself, challenges our pre-conceptions. A person with autism in the family alters the perspective; we are all more thoughtful, aware and empathic than before autism became a day-to-day reality for us.

My Grandson, Billy

by Richard Barber, Billy's Grandfather

Billy was a delightful, alert baby. Jon and Polly brought him with his older sister, Bella, to visit Kathy and me at our cottage on Tresco in the Isles of Scilly. Billy must have then been less than a year old and appeared completely normal. We had no idea of what was to come. We were just delighted that their small family seemed so happy and healthy.

Just over a year later, signs that Billy was no longer following the usual development path began to show themselves. Other members of our family, Polly's brother and sisters, for example, began to express concern about Billy. It was difficult to discuss it with Polly and Jon who, while accepting there was a problem, clung to any possibility other than autism. Maybe his speech problem was linked to a temporary deafness caused by glue-ear, maybe it was anything but autism.

Finally, the diagnosis was confirmed, and Polly and Jon accepted it. This was the point at which their characters were severely tested. All the family supported them and wanted to help in any way that we could. Polly's (and Jon's) concern for their child, Billy, was mirrored by my concern for my child, Polly. I felt that a heavy burden had been placed on her lovely, young family – now blessed with another son, Toby.

Jon and Polly's energy became supercharged. They took the attitude that nothing was incurable, even autism. If they could recover Billy's health, then perhaps thousands of other children could be helped as well.

Jon threw himself into researching everything about autism and followed up every avenue. Some were dead ends, but others showed dramatic results. Gradually, over a period of several years, Billy started to improve. Today he is a high-functioning child on the autism spectrum. Jon qualified as a nutritionist; Polly started an international magazine as a forum for professionals and parents of children with autism. She also created an international charity to provide a haven for adults with autism. Polly and Jon's lives have been changed. They have a driving energy and a belief that there are no boundaries to what can be achieved on behalf of families affected by autism.

And so Billy changed all of us. Like many people with autism, Billy is extraordinary. He has genius talents that lie hidden and which cannot be called upon at will. He views the world from his own private world into which we can scarcely venture. He will probably always need support, and yet he can give so much. He is a fascinating enigma, but above all he is a member of our family and we all love him.

What Jon and Polly have achieved for Billy they offer to all people dealing with autism through a magazine and a charity. As a family we offer love, support and practical help where we can. They began carrying a heavy burden and it soon became a crusade. Others joined and the burden became a little lighter. Like Polly, Jon and their friends, I believe that there is no limit to what we all can achieve for people with autism – and Billy is the inspiration.

I don't know if I believe in God, but I do believe in Good. A lot of Good has flowed from Billy's autism – and thus the world is a better place.

Autism in the Family

by Harriet, Polly's sister

I remember the news travelling around the family that Billy had been diagnosed as having 'autism'.

Straight away I felt for Polly, but I was initially taken aback by the response of various aunts that still thought it probably wasn't autism. This surprised me, as it was spoken with such certainty and reassurance by these well-meaning aunts. Their response of denial infuriated me, and was completely unhelpful, particularly when Polly needed family to listen to her and to then take on board what autism meant for Polly, Jon and Billy.

Polly would initially speak of Billy's sudden lack of eye

contact, communication and interest in others around him. These facts alone break my heart.

It's a terrible thing for a mother to be deprived of the key factors for communicating with her child. I cannot imagine how it must feel for a parent to reach out to their beloved son or daughter and always be unobserved or not properly noticed by their child. It feels like the worst punishment one could inflict on a mother who has an innate need to communicate easily with their child as if it were the most natural thing in the world. That is the point: it is, or should be, the most natural thing in the world – like breathing.

We should be able to take these qualities for granted.

With all these thoughts whirling round my head, I actually did little more than offer my sympathy to Polly by phone. I hardly saw Polly and her young family during the early years. I was a self-indulgent artist with no children of my own. I felt ill qualified to help out. I still feel guilty about this.

Now that I have children, I feel more tuned in to Polly and her daily challenges – I think. Actually, it's more that her experience as a mother of a child with autism has taught me to wonder about the environmental factors that surround us in general baby care. I think about the unnatural ingredients that surround us and our babies in modern society; for example, I am aware that it helps enormously to (when possible) keep babies and pregnant women away from contaminates such as artificial sweeteners, and toxic metals like mercury, or anything else that doesn't sit comfortably in a natural environment. After all, autism is a modern epidemic, so it is linked to modern life.

Billy's autism has made me sensitive to the delicateness of a growing baby's brain. One can easily imagine as one looks down at a new baby, how interfering with a baby's chemical and biological balance is a risky business. My driving instructor told me not to overtake if I was in any doubt. This 'If in doubt – don't!'

approach is one I take with my children's health when confronted with substances that just might threaten their development.

It is important to Polly that my children, who are of course blood-related to Billy, wouldn't be exposed to the same modern substances as Billy was in his first two years of life, particularly when his immune system was low, and then overloaded by an onslaught of environmental factors (in his case, antibiotics, cow's products like baby milk, and too many vaccinations).

I feel I owe thanks to Polly.

I have two 'healthy' daughters and that is partly due to Polly's interest in giving them the purest and cleanest start in life by keeping them away from possible contaminates that could threaten their natural development. She has taught me to use my common sense, logic, and our trusting instincts as mothers.

I still feel a little useless when it comes to making a difference to Billy, Polly and her family. This is partly due to Polly's generous personality; she expects nothing from people but seems to be always looking out for those around her.

Polly doesn't just cope: she started the *Autism File* magazine and The Autism Trust. This is on top of other big events like moving house and related projects.

In recent years I have been fortunate to be able to help with fundraising for The Autism Trust by donating my paintings to auction.

Polly recently remembered my harsh words clearly in our conversation when I found out that I had been diagnosed with breast cancer. I said, 'Well, I would rather be me, Polly, than you, taking my chances with breast cancer and knowing my children didn't have autism. You would want to swap with me if it meant that Billy no longer had autism.' I later apologised to Polly for being so brutal, and she said, 'No, Harriet, it was the right thing to admit.'

The most important thing to remember is that you are not alone
– none of us are. See our recommended sites and online groups
to join; they are full of wonderful parents, siblings and valuable
support.

In Part 2 we discuss the various approaches to education that
are available for children with autism and how to choose a school
that is right for your child.

PART 2

PROGRESSING THROUGH LEARNING

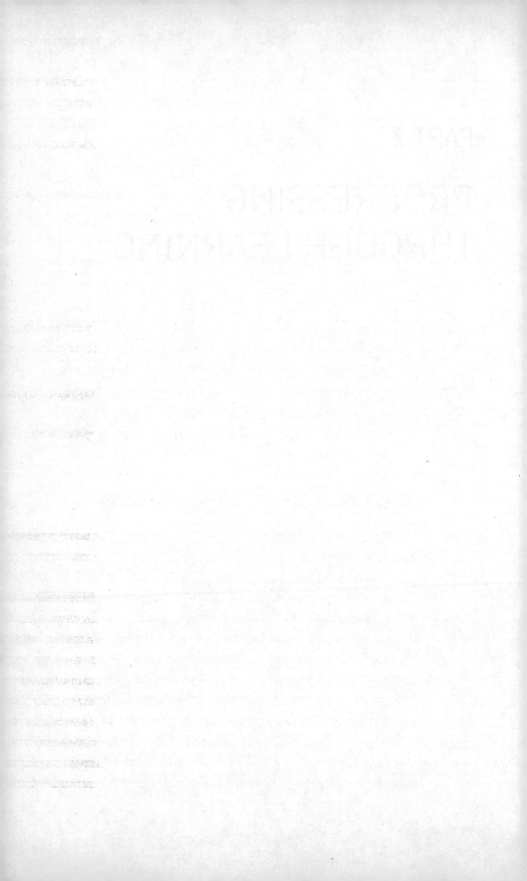

CHAPTER 7

Educational Approaches

Securing an ASC diagnosis for your child is likely to generate all manner of mixed feelings. On the one hand it will probably be something of a relief to have got to the end of a lengthy and fraught process furnished with a word you can use as shorthand to help other people understand what the issue is with your child. On the other hand you have had official confirmation that your child has a condition that could continue to affect him or her, and you, through life.

We are going to cover as many aspects as we can think of to do with finding and analysing the most effective education, therapy and support approaches for you and your child. This is obviously of vital importance to your child's development and your own peace of mind and can be hugely confusing if you're new to this.

Approaches to autism education

Choosing a suitable educational, therapeutic, behavioural or developmental approach to help your child is one of the most fraught and frustrating aspects of having a child with an ASC: you want to do what's best for your child, but you are faced with masses of complex and often contradictory information about the best way to go about it. For many of you, the most effective way forward in the medium term will be to find a suitable school, but this may yet be some time in the future and may then be complicated by the types of approach offered by any (relatively) local schools and by your own desire to seek the most effective strategy or combination of strategies to meet the specific needs of your own child.

The time between diagnosis and school placement (typically the two-plus years between two and a half and five), is a vital stage of your child's development and it is common sense to do what you can to capitalise on the potential gains to be had through early intervention while his or her brain is still developing rapidly and before behaviours become ingrained. Many of the independent treatment programmes available (often at a cost) are focused on early intervention with the aim of preparing your child to cope with the demands of mainstream schooling.

This chapter aims to give you an overview of the most widely used educational and therapeutic approaches and some insight into a select few of the vast range of intervention models available. The information we've provided here is for basic information only; you'll clearly want to do more of your own research, but this should demystify some of the named approaches you will have heard about.

ABA and Lovaas

What is ABA?

ABA is the application of the science of behaviourism to the treatment and education of children with special educational needs (SEN). In its most familiar form it is an intensive, one-to-one, home-based programme of skills training for children with autism and an ASC run by trained practitioners.

Applied behaviour analysis (ABA) does exactly what the name suggests: practitioners analyse a child's behaviour to determine the factors that contribute to that behaviour, and then apply the findings of this analysis to the practical modification of the behaviour. This can be to stop or reduce an undesirable behaviour, or to teach, reinforce or improve a desirable one. It used to be called 'behaviour modification'.

It's worth pointing out here that the word 'behaviour' doesn't necessarily refer to so-called autism behaviours or 'challenging' behaviours, but simply means any measurable action that the child can be observed doing; for example, giving eye contact in response to his or her name, touching an object on request, and so on.

What's the theory behind this approach?

The analysis of behaviour involves the detailed description of the 'ABC' – Antecedent (what happened prior to the behaviour), Behaviour (what the child actually does) and Consequences (what happens after, or as a result of the behaviour) in order to pin down the factors that motivate the child to perform in a certain way. Analysing this pattern allows practitioners to modify the consequences arising from specific antecedents and behaviours, which, when consistently applied, can gradually shape the child's responses.

In essence, ABA is based on the general principle that 'a behaviour that is rewarded is likely to be repeated' and involves the systematic reinforcement of desired behaviours through the use of rewards. When ABA first began to be used with people with learning difficulties, back in the 1960s and 1970s, the opposite of this principle was also applied – that is, undesirable behaviours were discouraged through the use of punishments or 'aversives', such as smacking and even electric shocks. These days, aversives are not used and undesirable or 'off-task' behaviours are addressed by ignoring them (thus denying the child the potentially motivating consequence of a reaction) or by withholding rewards and/or reinforcing and rewarding more desirable behaviours in their place.

What is the Lovaas method?

You might find this referred to variously as Lovaas ABA, The UCLA model of ABA, the Lovaas Programme, or EIBI, or others. (EIBI stands for Early Intensive Behavioural Intervention and is an umbrella term for various types of ABA approach including Lovaas and VB – see page 151.)

The Lovaas method uses 'discrete trial training' – repetitive one-to-one teaching sessions focused on a single behavioural outcome – measurable skills broken down into small steps and taught in a highly structured way. Based on the ABC model, each skill is delivered in intensive teaching sessions in a three-stage chain: (a) stimulus (an instruction or request; for example, 'pick up the ball'); (b) response (what the child does in response to the stimulus; for example, picks up the ball or not); and (c) consequence (a reward if the response is correct, or 'no' if incorrect). If the response is incorrect (as you would expect at the start of a new skill), the teacher will introduce a prompt, which could be anything from a further verbal instruction to (for example) directing the child's hand to the ball. If the response is correct, the child will be rewarded. Increasingly, ABA teachers use 'errorless teaching' methods, whereby minimal prompts are always used. In this way, the outcome is always successful (with support) and the motivating reward always forthcoming. Initially, rewards may be highly motivating tangible rewards such as small amounts of a favourite food (say, raisins or pieces of apple), a period of play with a favourite toy, and so on, but eventually these are phased out in favour of social rewards like verbal praise, hugs and tickles. The discrete trial is repeated many times in rapid succession, with a reward for each success and the gradual withdrawal of the prompt. (This is called 'fading'.)

The measurability of the child's behaviour is important and intrinsic to the science of behaviourism; in other words, only what is observable can properly be recorded. Thus, the outcomes of the 'trials' are focused on performable skills which demonstrate a desired level of understanding (feelings, thoughts, beliefs, and so on, are not observable, only actions).

The curriculum – that is, what skills are taught – is tailored to the individual needs of each child but based on a detailed developmental curriculum covering communication, attention, self-help, play, imitation and matching, world knowledge, and so on, as well as tackling 'maladaptive' (inappropriate) behaviours. The programme aims to teach basic skills and then to move on to more sophisticated language and social skills, as well as generalising learned skills to different situations.

The training programme usually consists of 30–40 hours of intensive work per week, delivered in the home by trained practitioners with structured consistency and the active involvement of parents (typically three to six people trained at the Lovaas Institute). This works out to 4–6 hours per day, 5–7 days a week for at least 2 years starting from as early an age as possible, with the aim of preparing the child for mainstream education wherever possible. The various studies carried out over the years by Lovaas and others emphasise the importance to the outcomes for the child of maintaining this intensity. Lovaas and his colleagues believe that the earlier the programme is started, the better the outcomes will be. He recommends starting before age three if possible and certainly before five. In practice, the average age to start the programme is about three and a half.

Where does it come from?

The application of ABA approaches to the treatment and education of children with autism is largely due to the work of Dr O. Ivar Lovaas, a clinical psychologist and psychology professor at UCLA (University of California at Los Angeles). Lovaas ABA is by no means the only dedicated ABA approach for children with autism, but it is the most widespread. Dr Lovaas began his work with older children by applying the principles of behavioural science and 'operant conditioning' developed by B. F. Skinner at Harvard (*Science and Human Behavior*, 1953). Lovaas had only limited success at the start, particularly as his clients were not able to maintain their skills once the treatment ended, except those whose parents followed up the work at home. He refined his approaches, concentrating on intensive, home-based treatment with children under five years and began to get more encouraging results. Through the mid 1960s and 1970s, Lovaas attracted a lot of criticism for his use of aversives but has subsequently developed alternative methods.

In 1981, Lovaas published *Teaching Developmentally Disabled Children: The Me Book*, which was a training manual for the application of behavioural therapy based on his work at UCLA. He published his initial experimental findings in 1987 and the approach has grown and flourished since then, becoming particularly popular in the UK and USA through the 1990s. Much of the popularity of the ABA approach in the 1990s was due to the success of the book *Let Me Hear your Voice: A Family's Triumph Over Autism* by Catherine Maurice, published in 1993. This was a moving account of a mother's attempts to help her two children who had autism and the success she had through the use of ABA approaches. Dr Maurice (Ph.D.) followed this up in 1996 with a very well-received manual called *Behavioural Intervention for Young Children with Autism: A Manual for Parents and Professionals.*

The Lovaas study (1987)

Lovaas's study ('Behavioral treatment and normal educational and intellectual functioning in young autistic children') was based on 61 children aged two to four years with an independent autism diagnosis and similar functioning levels, split into three groups: 19 in the experimental group and 21 in each of two control groups. The experimental group received 40 hours of intensive one-to-one ABA for at least two years, delivered in the home by UCLA psychology students trained and monitored by Lovaas. The first control group received only ten hours or less of the same programme and the second control group had no intervention from Lovaas's team (although some of the children in both control groups had other types of intervention).

The programme covered behavioural, social, cognitive and language deficits.

Findings

Of the 19 children in the experimental group, an average gain of 20 IQ points was attributed to the programme, whereas no discernible IQ gains were recorded for any of the children in the control groups. Nine of the 19 children (47 per cent) completed the first year of regular school following the intervention, and had measured IQs in the average to above average range, having gained an average of 30 IQ points since pre-programme testing. These nine were found to be 'normal-functioning' and were described as having 'recovered' from their autism.

Only one child from the 42 in the two control groups had a similar outcome.

Of the remaining ten children in the experimental group, eight were found to have made considerable gains in many areas, but still needed special schooling or additional support. The remaining two children were placed in specialist schools for children with autism or learning difficulties. In comparison, 53 per cent of the children in the control groups were placed in specialist autism or learning-difficulties schools.

A follow-up study of the nine children who made the most significant gains was conducted by Lovaas and his colleagues in 1993, based on data collected in the mid 1980s ('Long-term outcome for children with autism who received early intensive behavioral treatment').

One of the nine had subsequently been placed in a special education class, but another of the original 19 had come out of special Ed into mainstream. The children were tested for IQ, and also for life skills and social skills. All nine had retained the IQ gains they had made in the original study, and independent examiners were unable to distinguish them from their mainstream peers.

There have been some criticisms of the experimental methods used in Lovaas's studies, but overall it is accepted that the children did make significant gains which can be attributed directly to the ABA intervention, and similar results have been shown in subsequent studies.

CARD

The Center for Autism and Related Disorders (CARD) provides a variety of evidence-based treatment services to children with autism spectrum disorders (ASD). It was founded in Los Angeles in 1990 by Dr Doreen Granpeesheh.

What is it?

CARD treats children with a variety of diagnoses, including an ASC, PDD-NOS and Asperger's syndrome. The CARD Assessment Center provides behavioural, diagnostic and psychometric evaluations and assessments. Their specialised outpatient services clinic offers feeding intervention, medical treatment facilitation, and short-term intervention for severe behaviour. CARD's core service is early intensive behavioural intervention (EIBI), conducted within the client's home, school and community. Although the primary focus of CARD is EIBI, the CARD II programme treats individuals aged 8 to 21 years, concentrating on independent living, employment, leisure, friendship building and higher-education skills.

CARD provides comprehensive intervention programmes catered to each child's individual strengths and needs. They begin with a thorough evaluation and assessment of all areas of functioning. Challenging behaviours are assessed and parents are encouraged to seek full medical evaluations. The CARD curriculum is comprehensive and attends to all domains of functioning, including language, play, social, motor, academic, adaptive, cognitive and executive functioning skills. Over 3000 lessons make up the CARD curriculum, and programmes are grounded on age-appropriate norms based on typical child development. The increasing demand for CARD services and the need for worldwide dissemination of ABA has led to the development of SKILLS (shaping knowledge through individualised life learning systems), an online training, assessment, programme design and progress-tracking system, built around the CARD curriculum.

CARD is also dedicated to research in ASCs. Faculty in the CARD research and development department have authored over 70 publications related to autism, behaviour analysis, and other topics in psychology. Over the past 20 years, CARD has become a leading provider of behavioural intervention and has effectively treated thousands of children with an ASC. CARD believes in recovery from an ASC, and they have witnessed recovery in a significant number of their clients. Although recovery is still not possible for the majority of children with an ASC, CARD endeavours to make every child reach his or her maximum potential, whatever that may be. CARD is dedicated to providing the highest quality behavioural intervention to the greatest number of children with an ASC around the world.

Verbal behaviour approach (VB)

The verbal behaviour approach has become popular in recent years due to its focus on the application of ABA approaches to functional language development. This approach goes back to B.F. Skinner's original analysis of verbal behaviour in the 1950s ('Verbal behaviour', 1957) as interpreted by Drs Mark Sundberg and James Partington in two seminal publications in 1998: *Assessment of Basic Language and Learning Skills* and *Teaching Language to Children with Autism and Other Developmental Disabilities*.

What is it?

VB sets out to teach and reinforce spoken language by linking it to meaning. The child is taught to use language to communicate rather than just to label objects or imitate sounds.

Although VB shares much of the organisation and structure of Lovaas's method, including discrete trials and rewards, and employs the errorless teaching method, it differs from the Lovaas approach to language acquisition in a couple of significant areas. Firstly, VB is much more focused on 'functional' language – it concentrates on a rounded use and generalised understanding of language concepts – whereas the Lovaas approach tends to see language development as a linear developmental progression from receptive to expressive language. In simple terms, Lovaas sets out to teach language skills from a developmental curriculum, whereas VB focuses on what the child wants and sets out to teach him how to request it (a similar approach to PECS, page 161, though by different means). VB also concentrates on learning in the child's natural environment (NET – natural environment training) rather than in the rather more rarefied and structured conditions of the discrete trials in Lovaas's model.

TEACCH

What is it?

Treatment and Education of Autistic and related Communication-handicapped Children (TEACCH) is an evidence-based, structured teaching approach set up originally in the 1970s by Eric Schopler, Ph.D., in the Department of Psychiatry at the University of North Carolina and now part of the Carolina Institute for Developmental Disabilities. Division TEACCH runs a comprehensive programme for people with an ASC throughout North Carolina, but outside the state (for example, in the UK), rather than being a self-contained programme, TEACCH is a set of principles and strategies that can be applied across a range of settings.

TEACCH is the most widely used (named) approach in UK

schools, although is likely to take different forms in different settings due to the fact that it constitutes an approach and a philosophy rather than a packaged programme or curriculum.

In addition to its own state-wide programmes, Division TEACCH – the established centre for the advancement and dissemination of this approach – is also noted for its extensive training and research activities.

The TEACCH 'structured teaching' approach is notable for its emphasis on modifying and structuring the environment to accommodate the specific strengths and deficits of people with an ASC; what TEACCH calls 'the culture of autism', and on tailoring structured programmes to the individual needs of each person, continually updated by regular assessment. It also puts a high value on presenting tasks and challenges visually so as to address the issues arising from the difficulties people with an ASC face with regard to social communication, reciprocal social interaction and imaginative thought processes (the triad of impairments), and on promoting the role of parents as co-therapists.

Typically, a TEACCH programme will involve the organisation of uncluttered (distraction-free) workspaces, the separation of distinct areas in the room for different activities, the use of individualised personal schedules, the organisation of tasks using pictures and symbols, tasks and activities presented in a left-to-right sequence, objects, rooms, storage and resources, and so on, clearly labelled. Teachers will put a lot of emphasis on the specific needs of individuals, the way an ASC affects them, the things that motivate them (both social and tangible rewards, or 'reinforcers', are used), the way that individuals learn, etc. Effectively, the environment and teaching approaches are contrived to be understandable and navigable to people with autism in a way that promotes development and independence. The TEACCH website (www.teacch.com) puts it as follows:

The long-term goals of the TEACCH approach are both skill development and fulfilment of fundamental human needs, such as dignity, engagement in productive and personally meaningful activities, and feelings of security, self-efficacy and self-confidence. To accomplish these goals, TEACCH developed the intervention approach called Structured Teaching.

The principles of Structured Teaching include:

- Understanding the culture of autism.
- Developing an individualised person- and family-centred plan for each client or student, rather than using a standard curriculum.
- Structuring the physical environment.
- Using visual supports to make the sequence of daily activities predictable and understandable.
- Using visual supports to make individual tasks understandable.

What's the theory behind this approach?

TEACCH is based on principles of cognitive social learning theory (sometimes called social cognitive theory and predominantly the work of Bandura and Walters, 1963) which asserts that it is cognitive features – aspects of thinking, such as expectation, situational understanding and 'meaningfulness' – rather than reward and punishment that shape and determine an individual's learning and responses to environmental forces (although they also play a part). TEACCH was therefore devised as a way of thinking about the patterns of thinking, learning and behaviour in autism and emphasises expectation and the establishment of meaningfulness in a given situation so as to help the person with an ASC to understand the bigger picture, rather than simply relying on training responses for reward.

In addition, TEACCH also uses principles of developmental psychology in that activities and experiences are presented at levels commensurate with the child's developmental level, again so as to promote maximum understanding. For this reason, TEACCH advocates continuous assessment of skill acquisition and developmental progress as a vital prerequisite for programme planning.

The 'Culture of Autism' is central to the TEACCH philosophy and continually refers practitioners back to the specificity of how autism affects that individual, so as to organise the visual environment, resources, instructions, and so on, accordingly. This is how Division TEACCH defines the Culture of Autism:

- Relative strength in, and preference for, processing visual information (compared to difficulties with auditory processing, particularly of language).
- Frequent attention to details but difficulty understanding the meaning of how those details fit together.
- Difficulty combining ideas.
- Difficulty with organising ideas, materials and activities.
- Difficulties with attention. (Some individuals are very distractible; others have difficulty shifting attention when it's time to make transitions.)
- Communication problems, which vary by developmental level but always include impairments in the social use of language (called 'pragmatics').
- Difficulty with concepts of time, including moving too quickly or too slowly and having problems recognising the beginning, middle or end of an activity.
- Tendency to become attached to routines, with the result that activities may be difficult to generalise from the original learning situation, and disruptions in routines can be upsetting, confusing or uncomfortable.
- Very strong interests and impulses to engage in favoured activities, with difficulties disengaging once engaged.
- Marked sensory preferences and dislikes.

Although they are both structured approaches, unlike ABA, TEACCH believes that the type of structure inherent in discrete trial training is likely to lead to 'prompt dependence', thus compounding the existing difficulty that people with an ASC have in generalising skills from one situation to another. Its structure is therefore built into the environment, to make it accessible to the child.

Where does it come from?

TEACCH has grown and developed over 40 years from the work of Eric Schopler. As a post-graduate student at the University of Chicago, Schopler had studied under Bruno Bettelheim. Bettelheim's rather extreme views (now widely discredited) that autism arose in children due to feelings of hostility and rejection caused by emotionally cold parents ('refrigerator mothers') caused Schopler to reject contemporary perceptions of autism as a mental illness, concluding that this widely held view, and the 'scapegoating' of parents, was ill-informed, counterproductive and arose out of frustration at the lack of empirical knowledge on the true nature of the condition. He therefore set out to study autism through empirical research and the application of other significant psychological theories in order to develop an effective approach to treatment and education.

The TEACCH programme has emerged and developed as a direct result of the findings of Schopler's research, along with colleagues – notably Robert Reichler and Gary Mesibov.

The Son-Rise Program

What is it?

The Son-Rise Program® is a home-based, child-centred one-to-one programme for people with autism, an ASC, Asperger's syndrome and PDD-NOS, run by parents and volunteers who are trained in specific types of interactions with their child through courses run by The Autism Treatment Center of America:

The Son-Rise Program® teaches a specific and comprehensive system of treatment and education designed to help families and caregivers enable their children to dramatically improve in all areas of learning, development, communication and skill acquisition. It offers highly effective educational techniques, strategies and principles for designing, implementing and maintaining a stimulating, high-energy, one-on-one, home-based, child-centered program.

Son-Rise is based on the principle that the 'social and relational' deficit of autism underlies all other aspects (for example, communication, inflexibility, and so on) and that only by completely loving and accepting your child, and capitalising on his or her own motivations can you build a relationship that will help them to grow and change, with the stated possibility of full or partial recovery from autism.

The core programme involves 'joining' enthusiastically with your child in their repetitive or ritualistic behaviours within a structured environment (typically a specially set-up and structured playroom), so as to create a relationship over time based on what motivates them, rather than imposing conformity to a set of rules or types of behaviour they don't yet understand. Once the relationship starts to become established and interaction becomes more frequent and more meaningful, it is then possible to use the child's own particular interests to guide them, through interactive play, towards social and developmental goals.

What's the theory behind this approach?

Son-Rise sees the recognisable features of autism as an understandable response to the child's disordered perception of the world. This is based on an understanding of autism that acknowledges a basis in altered neurological development and emphasises the significance of an underlying sensory integration disorder.

Son-Rise principles are built on certain assertions about autism, which can be defined as follows:

- Children with autism have an underlying sensory integration disorder. This affects their ability to process sensory information – what they see, hear, touch, taste and smell, and so on – in order to filter out and focus on what might be considered the important bits.

  This means, for instance, that the ticking of the clock or the dog barking in the distance can have as much impact, volume and significance in their disordered perception as does the sound of their mother's voice.

  The same could be true of visual senses, the objects, lights and colours in the environment competing for significance with people's faces, or of tactile sensations, a light touch perhaps being perceived as if it were as invasive and unpleasant as a pinch, particularly where the child cannot predict or comprehend the reason for the touch.

- Children with autism are therefore completely overwhelmed and stressed by the onslaught of unfiltered sensory input, by the consequent unpredictability of the world around them and by the harmful effects of stress hormones (for example, cortisol and epinephrine).

  Our own ability to constantly filter and organise sensory input is what enables us to learn what things do, why they're there, how some things interact with other things and therefore to be able to predict or anticipate what might happen in any given situation.

  If the neural pathways that enable the exchange of information between parts of the brain are dysfunctional, or not properly constructed through typical learning and development, this impairs the child's ability to 'compute' the relationship of one piece of information to another and leaves them unable to assign priorities for their attention, or to predict actions or outcomes.

- The most significant source of sensory overload and unpredictability to children with autism is the actions and interactions of other people, particularly as this will tend to be thrust upon them, and may be focused on making the child do something other than what they've chosen to do.

  Given the implications of the above information on sensory perception, the demands of 'social' engagement are likely to be perceived by the child as noisy, confusing and invasive.

- The child understandably develops patterns of behaviour that enable him or her to 'tune out' the overwhelming sensory overload and unpredictability of the world around them by tuning in to familiar or predictable activities such as repetitive physical mannerisms and rituals, pattern-making (lining things up), 'obsessive preoccupations' or special interests, and so on.

  Son-Rise does not believe that repetitive mannerisms are necessarily self-stimulatory and refers to these as 'isms', rather than 'stimming'. (Stimming is a repetitive body movement designed to stimulate one or more of the senses. The term is shorthand for self-stimulation. It manifests itself in many different ways, but is often exemplified by the flapping of hands, spinning, rocking and so on.)

It is clearly important when investigating any programme or treatment to do as much research as possible, so the following information should be considered alongside all the other information and explanation offered by The Autism Treatment Center.

  The website lists how the programme benefits children with special needs:

- Joining in a child's repetitive and ritualistic behaviours supplies the key to unlocking the mystery of these behaviours and facilitates eye contact, social development and the inclusion of others in play.

- Utilising a child's own motivation advances learning and builds the foundation for education and skill acquisition.
- Teaching through interactive play results in effective and meaningful socialisation and communication.
- Using energy, excitement and enthusiasm engages the child and inspires a continuous love of learning and interaction.
- Employing a non-judgmental and optimistic attitude maximises the child's enjoyment, attention and desire throughout their Son-Rise Program.
- Placing the parent as the child's most important and lasting resource provides a consistent and compelling focus for training, education and inspiration.
- Creating a safe, distraction-free work–play area facilitates the optimal environment for learning and growth.

Where does it come from?

The approach that became the Son-Rise Program was initially devised by Barry and Samahria Kaufman in the 1970s to help their own son, Raun, who was diagnosed with severe autism having developed normally until the age of 13–14 months. He then regressed, lost his previous language and social skills, and presented typical autistic features such as spinning objects and flapping his hands; he had very little eye contact and no language. The Kaufmans were told that Raun's condition was hopeless and lifelong and that he should be institutionalised.

Rejecting this prognosis, the Kaufmans devised their own home-based programme to reach their supposedly unreachable child. After three and a half years of intensive work, Raun was fully recovered, had a successful mainstream education and is now the CEO of The Autism Treatment Center of America. Based on their success with their own son, and with the book they wrote about their story, the Kaufmans founded the Options Institute in 1983 and have been offering the Son-Rise Program to help children, parents and professionals ever since.

PECS

What is it?

The Picture Exchange Communication System (PECS) is an 'augmentative' communication system that teaches children with autism (and other social and communication disorders) to communicate spontaneously by exchanging picture symbols. The emphasis of this approach is on teaching language-impaired children to initiate communication in order to have their needs met, rather than simply responding to prompts from others.

It is important to distinguish between augmentative and alternative communication systems. An alternative system, like sign language, is designed to take the place of spoken language, whereas an augmentative communication system, such as PECS, is designed to be used to accompany and enhance (that is, augment) spoken language. The issue that PECS has been developed to address is not necessarily difficulties in the mechanics of expressive language, but rather the complexities of functional, social language use. Although the main aim of PECS is to promote the development of communication rather than of speech, it has contributed significantly to the development of spoken language in many children, as it helps to overcome functional and structural issues.

Children using PECS are taught to approach an adult spontaneously (social approach) and hand over a picture of something they want in exchange for the item. In this way, the communication of the child's needs is not dependent on prompts from the adult or on imitation, etc., but is a deliberate act of 'communicative intent' within a social context. In addition, the act of exchange incorporates the interactive element of communication, the giving of a thought to another person, whereas signing, pointing to pictures and even spoken words can be delivered without necessarily engaging with the other person.

Key to the success of the PECS approach to communication training is that the child must be motivated to communicate. It is therefore vital in the initial stage (phase 1) that the picture symbol used in the first phase of training represents something that the child really wants, and that the request is honoured immediately. So the process starts with the trainer figuring out with the child what is most motivating – that is, what they most desire. The desired item is the reward or 'reinforcer' and the child is taught in a highly structured way to exchange the picture for the item.

In subsequent phases of the programme, children are taught to seek out adults to exchange, to discriminate between pictures and select the one they want, to construct sentences with pictures, respond to questions, comment on their surroundings and then to build up their vocabulary with simple adjectives (colours, sizes, and so on).

What's the theory behind this approach?

The development of PECS is essentially based on a considered response to, and refinement of, existing approaches using pictures and symbols that stem from the widely accepted assertion (supported by a good deal of research evidence) that children with autism process visual information considerably better than they process auditory information, and that many of the difficulties they have with communication arise from the social function rather than the mechanics.

The developers assert that other approaches that were prevalent at the time, such as sign language, picture-point systems and speech training, are limited in their effectiveness because they miss this vital functional, spontaneous and interactive element.

Where does it come from?

PECS was developed in 1985 by clinical psychologist Andy Bondy, Ph.D., and speech and language therapist Lori Frost, MS.CCC/ SLP, as part of an ABA-based education programme, The Pyramid Approach to Education, which combines ABA with functional approaches. The Pyramid Approach and PECS originated in the USA (Newark, New Jersey), but now has centres worldwide, including in the UK (Brighton).

Social Stories

What is it?

Social Stories is a way of teaching social skills and social understanding to children with an ASC, particularly in situations they may otherwise find confusing, difficult or distressing. Stories are developed to address specific issues with individuals and aim to help the child to interpret otherwise 'hidden' social cues and meanings so as to understand and cope better with the situation.

Social Stories is a clear description in writing of the key elements of a given situation, describing factual details about what is happening, what might happen, what things are for, and so on, along with social elements, such as what others might be expecting, what the young person could do, how others might respond and why.

Once constructed, the story can be read through by the child with or without support to remind him or her of the issues and possible solutions.

Social Stories, as defined by its creator, Carol Gray, are constructed according to a particular format, written as if from the child's point of view in the first person and present tense. The format should include:

- **Descriptive sentences**. These are who, what, where, when and why statements, describing factual elements of the situation; for example, 'I go to school on the school bus. On some days the bus arrives before 8.00, on other days the bus arrives after 8.00. When the bus arrives after 8.00 it still takes me to school.'

- **Perspective sentences**. These describe how the people involved might react to the same situation; for example,

'Sometimes I get worried if the bus does not arrive before 8.00. Mum and Dad don't get worried; they know the bus will come. Mum and Dad don't like it when I get upset.'

- **Directive sentences**. These offer an approach to the child as to how he or she might cope with the situation; for example, 'I will try hard to stay calm if the bus doesn't arrive before 8.00. I will try to wait quietly.'

- **Control sentences**. Created by the child with support and only usually applicable to higher functioning children, these describe strategies that he or she can use to work through the situation and remember the important bits; for example, 'If the bus doesn't arrive by 8.00, I can go to the front window, and then I know I'll see the bus when it arrives.'

Other sentence types can also be included in the story according to the needs and abilities of the individual and the specifics of the situation.

In general terms, and obviously depending on the ability of the child, the descriptive and perspective sentences should outweigh directive sentences, giving as much information as possible about the context and social ramifications of the situation. Depending on the particular needs, abilities or learning styles of the child, Social Stories can be constructed equally effectively using symbols, photographs, objects, dolls, tape recordings or role play on video, and so on.

Comic Strip Conversations

Along the same lines as Social Stories, Comic Strip Conversations aims to furnish a child with information about the key elements of a situation. In this case, the situation is typically a conversation or interaction between two or more people. Comic Strip Conversations sets out to use simple drawings, speech bubbles, thought bubbles and colour to help the child to understand the dynamics of conversation by illustrating what people say, what they mean and what they might be thinking.

What's the theory behind this approach?

The development of Social Stories and Comic Strip Conversations was based to a large extent on the deficit in reciprocal social interaction defined within the triad of impairments and on the complex issues for people with an ASC arising from their difficulties with interpreting the thoughts, motivations, opinions, plans, wishes and expectations of others, as described by the 'theory of mind' (see box).

Where does it come from?

Social Stories and Comic Book Conversations were devised in 1991 by Carol Gray, a special-education teacher and consultant for children and adults with autism and an ASC and now director of the Gray Center for Social Learning and Understanding in Grand Rapids, Michigan.

Theory of mind

Theory of mind describes the ability to attribute mental states (such as beliefs, wishes, plans, opinions and emotions) to yourself or others and to understand that other people's mental states may be different from your own. There is a large amount of research data (particularly by Simon Baron-Cohen, Francesca Happé and others) to support the assertion that people with autism have distinct and significant deficits in theory of mind, and that this is not necessarily related to intelligence level and is therefore a specific deficit attributable to the condition of autism/ASC.

Cognitive, social and perceptual problems arising from deficits in theory of mind have been found to be wide ranging in people with an ASC compared to typically developing children and children with developmental disorders other than autism.

The classic example is a false-belief task, often called the 'Sally Anne task'. In this task the child is shown a simple story, acted out with two dolls, Sally and Anne. Sally has a basket and Anne has a box. Sally also has a marble, which she puts in her basket. Sally then goes away for a while. While Sally is away, Anne takes the marble from the basket and puts it in the box. Sally then comes back.

Having watched all this happen, the child is then asked, 'Where will Sally look for her marble?'

Children who have a theory of mind will know that Sally doesn't know that the marble was moved and surmise that she will look in the basket for it. A child whose theory of mind is impaired or absent will answer that Sally will look in the box, i.e. where the child knows the marble to be. They are not able to separate their own perceptions from Sally's and will not understand that Sally has her own beliefs that may not be accurate.

Studies have shown that the majority (up to 80 per cent in some studies) of children with an ASC cannot pass this test. Even children with high-functioning autism and Asperger's syndrome who, by definition, have an IQ within the normal range, cannot pass the test until years after their non-autistic peers.

This is a classic and oft-quoted test, but theory of mind goes a long way beyond this. It not only affects children's ability to interpret what others think in a given situation as opposed to what they themselves think but it also affects their ability to detect when or if a person is thinking by their eye-gaze or behaviour. Furthermore, it affects their ability to determine when others are joking, lying, pretending or being sarcastic, as perceiving this would require them to understand that the intentions of the other person might be at odds with the words spoken or actions taken.

Therapeutic approaches

It's actually quite difficult to separate educational approaches from therapeutic approaches, as there is a high degree of overlap and they're all focused on enhancing learning and development in various ways; however, the following clutch of interventions call themselves therapies and tend to be used to augment education and promote well-being and development in emotional and sensory domains. You will find versions of many of these therapeutic interventions being used in schools as highly valued strategies alongside more traditional teaching methods or as part of a combination of approaches.

Intensive Interaction Therapy (IIT)

What is it?

Intensive interaction is a practical, pleasurable, free-flowing approach to teaching and guiding the development of non-verbal communication and social skills to people with autism and/or severe and complex learning difficulties. It can also be seen simply as a way to be with people, enriching interactions and promoting shared enjoyment in each other's company.

Intensive interaction focuses on the concepts and skills that precede the development of speech or accompany early stages of language development. These are known as the Fundamentals of Communication. The approach has been developed for use with people with severe and profound learning disabilities, but is applicable to those who may have more advanced language skills or higher functioning levels but are uncommunicative or extremely socially isolated.

The interactions are non-directive in that the therapist (parent or caregiver) does not work to a set agenda, but follows the lead of the child: responding to what they do, commenting on their actions, laughing, imitating or mirroring their movements, using gesture, posture, body language, facial expression, and responding to the person's sounds and actions as if they were meaningful communication. The skill of the therapist is in enhancing and promoting the fun and reciprocity of the communicative exchange and modifying volume, intensity, pace, proximity, and so on, so as to remain non-invasive, non-threatening and a good communication partner.

The Fundamentals of Communication in their simplest form are listed in various media as follows:

- Enjoying being with another person.
- Developing the ability to attend to that person.
- Concentration and attention span.
- Learning to do sequences of activity with the other person.
- Taking turns in exchanges of behaviour.
- Sharing personal space.
- Using and understanding eye contacts.
- Using and understanding facial expressions.
- Using and understanding physical contacts.
- Using and understanding non-verbal communication.
- Vocalisations, extending the range of vocalisations and using vocalisations with meaning.
- Complicated emotional learning – bonding, empathy, understanding other people, and so on.

Intensive interaction has been found to be effective in promoting the development of communicative and interactive behaviours such as eye-contact, shared attention, smiling, vocalising, initiating social contact, communicating needs and preferences, making and imitating sounds, gestures, and so on.

What's the theory behind this approach?

IIT is influenced by a huge body of research evidence about the way that children develop language, communication and social skills in the first year of life.

This is an intense and rapid period of learning and development in the extraordinarily complex and sophisticated fundamentals of communication, conversation and socialisation and is conducted in a non-directive, unstructured and unsystematic way.

The psychologist Geraint (Gary) Ephraim, Ph.D., developed theoretical approaches to working with people with severe learning difficulties based on the understanding of early development and infant/caregiver interactions. He argued that adults with learning disabilities needed to learn fundamental communication and social abilities in a naturalistic way, through the kind of interactive play that babies and parents do. He called this approach 'augmented mothering'.

Where does it come from?

Intensive interaction as we know it today was developed and pioneered in the mid 1980s by Dave Hewett, and Melanie Nind, a headteacher and teacher working with people at the Harperbury Hospital School, in Hertfordshire, UK, who had severe learning difficulties, most of whom were unable to communicate verbally, and many of whom had autism diagnoses.

Hewett and Nind, along with other staff at the school, were dissatisfied with the prevalent behavioural and skill-based models of teaching and interaction and began to experiment with different ways of building relationships and interacting with their extremely socially isolated learners.

Influenced by the work and ideas of Gary Ephraim, research on early communication and their own relevant experience, Hewett and Nind developed the intensive interaction approach, incorporating their own academic study to focus on the Fundamentals of Communication, on how children learn to be communicators and on joining the children 'in their own world' rather than imposing structure from outside.

Sensory Integration Therapy

What is it?

Sensory Integration Therapy is a programme of movements, experiences and exercises designed to improve sensory processing. It is typically offered as a therapeutic approach within the remit of trained occupational therapists.

Sensory integration refers to the processing in the brain and central nervous system of information gathered by the senses from the environment and from the body itself in order to organise it, interpret it and respond appropriately. These processes are essential to understanding and learning about the world, to the establishment of strong neural connections in the brain and to the development of self-image and the regulation of behaviour.

Many people with autism have difficulties associated with the processing of sensory information, leading either to hypersensitivity (oversensitivity) or hyposensitivity (undersensitivity) to sensory stimuli like light, sound, touch, and so on. These problems are often referred to as 'sensory integration dysfunction' or 'sensory processing disorder' although these are not formal diagnoses.

Most people process sensory information automatically, and naturally develop discrimination and tolerances within each sense, such as recognition of comparative brightness, volume, lightness of touch, and so on.

People with sensory integration difficulties experience sensory input in a different way and can develop various hypersensitive or hyposensitive reactions and associated behaviours. These may include things like experiencing sounds or colours as painful or intolerable, rejecting physical contact or removing clothing, developing strange postures, spinning and jumping around or being sluggish and poorly coordinated. Each of these behaviours (and many others) may indicate a disordered sensory perception and may be addressed through Sensory Integration Therapy.

Sensory Integration Therapy usually consists of guiding the child through a series of specialised exercises and sensory experiences, often in a special sensory room equipped with a variety of balance boards, exercise balls, barrels, swings, hammocks and often moving lights, bubble tubes and music players.

Occupational therapists offering sensory integration will often also develop programmes of sensory integration to be followed at home, including recommending particular toys, foods, physical organisation of spaces, to exercise or regulate sensory input. The aim is to help the child to learn to regulate their own sensory responses and tolerances, in order to cope better with the world.

What's the theory behind this approach?

No one is entirely sure why so many children with autism experience sensory difficulties, although some believe that it is due to differences in brain structure and neural growth, possibly related to the onset of autism affecting the natural investigation of and interaction with people and with the environment that is vital to neural growth.

Where does it come from?

Sensory Integration Theory and Sensory Integration Therapy were developed by occupational therapist and clinical psychologist Dr A. Jean Ayres, Ph.D. OTR, in the 1970s, while on the faculty of the University of Southern California (USC).

Difficulties arising from disordered sensory perception

Within each of the senses, children with disordered sensory processing may develop hyper- or hyposensitivities. Hypersensitivity means oversensitivity and is likely to lead to avoidance (of loud noises, touch and bright lights). Hyposensitivity means undersensitivity and often results in actively seeking extreme sensory experiences in order to compensate.

In the chart overleaf are a few examples of ways these could present themselves.

Sense	Hyper (avoider)	Hypo (seeker)
Sight	Avoids bright lights, eye contact; doesn't like certain colours	Stares at people or objects; 'examines' objects closely; likes spinning or sparkly objects
Hearing	Puts fingers in ears; reacts adversely to seemingly mundane or distant sounds	Seems not to notice loud or intrusive noises; talks too loudly or makes shrill noises
Touch *	Rejects physical contact; finds clothing uncomfortable; doesn't like messy play	Touches objects and surfaces all the time; always gets dirty, doesn't notice dirty hands or face
Taste	Very 'faddy' with food; rejects certain foods; likes bland foods	Seeks strong flavours; eats non-food items
Smell	More sensitive to certain odours; may be put off certain foods	Sniffs and smells people and objects
Vestibular	Doesn't like being upside down; avoids jumping and climbing activities or uneven surfaces; doesn't like heights	Spins self without getting dizzy; very physically active and fidgety; never seems to tire

Sense	Hyper (avoider)	Hypo (seeker)
Proprioception	May be clumsy and uncoordinated; can't catch a ball	Likes tight clothing; seeks rough and tumble; likes to be squashed in small spaces; hits or pushes too hard, etc.; may bite nails or chew things

* The final two are generally included under 'touch', but issues in these specific areas may still be familiar

Temperature	Feels the cold; puts on too many clothes	Happy in short sleeves when it's really cold
Pain	Seems to experience a light touch as if painful; hates hair brushing and towelling	Doesn't seem to feel pain; doesn't respond badly to injury, injections, etc.

Massage and aromatherapy

What is it?

Massage therapy and aromatherapy are separate therapeutic approaches, but are often combined because, in addition to the independent benefits of both therapies, massage is a very efficient way of introducing essential oils to the body, which, as I explain below, are beneficial to the body and mind. Both approaches are considered beneficial and effective aids to relaxation and stress-reduction for people with an ASC, but can also be stimulating and invigorating as required.

Massage is the manipulation of the soft tissues of the body (skin, muscles, tendons and ligaments), improving circulation and helping the transportation of oxygen and nutrients to body tissues, relieving pain, soreness and stiffness in muscles and improving flexibility.

Aromatherapy is the therapeutic use of aromatic essential oils – concentrated extracts derived from trees and plants, to stimulate specific physiological and emotional responses in the brain and body through the sense of smell.

In addition to the introduction of essential oils through aromatherapy massage, oils can be used in a variety of ways, such as in a room spray, warmed in a diffuser, or applied to a tissue, pillow or soft toy.

The dedicated programmes TouchTalks and Aromacare have been specially designed to deliver accredited training in massage and aromatherapy in a range of care and education settings (including at home), and were devised within an ASC setting for parents and practitioners. TouchTalks introduces caregivers to the fundamentals of calming, relaxing and non-invasive massage, and Aromacare combines similar strategies, plus more advanced massage, with the most effective elements of aromatherapy.

Both training programmes are particularly applicable to supporting calming, self-control and relaxation for people with an ASC and are accredited by the International Federation of Aromatherapists.

What's the theory behind this approach?

Neither massage therapy nor aromatherapy is an intervention specifically designed or adapted for the treatment of people with an ASC, but both have been shown to be beneficial, particularly in the management and amelioration of stress, anxiety, depression and mood disorders.

People with an ASC are known to be particularly vulnerable to stress and high levels of anxiety, and this is widely believed to be at the root of many mood disorders and behavioural difficulties due to complex issues arising from the social and cognitive demands of everyday life. A number of disorders can be greatly eased through massage: muscular tension, poor muscle tone, low energy, stiffness and inflexibility, elevated heart rate, rapid breathing and many other side effects of stress, as well as poor digestion, poor nutrition and insufficient exercise. The physical contact inherent in massage can be highly effective in calming and in developing interpersonal relationships.

Aromatherapy is based on the widely experienced, but little-understood, power of the sense of smell. This is rooted in the molecular science of olfaction as it affects mental states, now known as aromachology.

Smell is an extraordinarily sophisticated chemical analysis of odour molecules as they pass through the nose and are interpreted by the part of the brain (the limbic system) that also manages memory, mood and emotion. Different plant extracts have different chemical effects. They connect with different, finely tuned receptors and stimulate certain neurotransmitters in the brain (such as serotonin) that affect mood, emotional response and mental state.

Where does it come from?

The therapeutic use of aromatic herbs dates back many thousands of years and has been a part of many cultures' medicinal practices ever since. In more modern times, a French chemist and perfumier, in the 1880s, called René-Maurice Gattefossé, is credited with the re-discovery of the therapeutic qualities of essential oils and with coining the term *aromatherapie*. His work was later picked up by a succession of doctors and biochemists, particularly a French doctor called Jean Valnet who used essential oils to treat gangrene during the Second World War and was the first to use aroma to address psychiatric conditions, and an

Austrian biochemist named Madame Marguerite Maury who published a book on the subject in France in 1961. The first major work in English, *The Art of Aromatherapy*, was published by Robert Tisserand in 1977 and is still considered the most influential reference on the subject.

Often considered the oldest form of therapy, massage dates back to at least 3000 BC in China and was widely used by the Greek civilisation. Its history is far too long and involved to detail here, but the type of massage generally used today, often known as 'Swedish massage' is credited to a Dutchman named Johann Mezger, who introduced the techniques to the medical establishment and first used the French terms *effleurage*, *petrissage* and *tapotement* that are still used by practitioners today to describe different types of massage stroke.

Music therapy

What is it?

Music therapy is a widely used therapeutic intervention that uses guided music-making and improvisation, rhythm, song and musical games to stimulate meaningful relationships, social communication, language skills and emotional expression. Individual music therapy is provided charitably by some organisations or in association with some schools, LEAs or health trusts and is available privately.

What's the theory behind this approach?

Music is able to create interest and emotional responses in people without involving verbal or overt social interaction and is a non-threatening way to introduce and develop skills of interaction, turn-taking, call and response, and other valuable pre-verbal language and social skills to people with an ASC. The rhythms, structures and modulations of music, along with its virtually universal appeal, make it an ideal tool for building therapeutic relationships.

Music therapy has been shown to be effective with some children with an ASC in improving communicative and social behaviour, developing an outlet for emotional expression, reducing self-stimulatory or acting-out behaviours and improving concentration.

Where does it come from?

The therapeutic use of music to influence health, well-being and even behaviour dates right back to ancient civilisations, but music therapy as we know it today is generally thought to have emerged during the First World War as a treatment for trauma victims. The two most widely used approaches in the UK – Nordoff Robbins music therapy and analytical music therapy – emerged from the work of Paul Nordoff and Clive Robbins through the 1950s and 1960s, and Juliette Alvin and Mary Priestly in the 1960s and 1970s.

Higashi (Daily Life Therapy)

What is it?

Daily Life Therapy is sometimes known as the 'Higashi method' from the name of the school where it originated – Higashi means 'hope'. It is a school-based educational philosophy developed in the 1960s and 1970s by Dr Kiyo Kitahara, specifically for children with autism, based on daily exercise, strict routines and regimented learning. As such, the Higashi method is actually more educational than therapeutic, and was once the big buzz in autism education.

What's the theory behind this approach?

The approach aims to promote self-identity and independence through vigorous and regular physical exercise and regimented teaching methods based on highly structured rote learning and imitating tasks in groups, in an integrated school setting.

The curriculum focuses on self-care skills (for daily life) and independence, as well as an academic and arts-based curriculum, supported by the three fundamental 'pillars' of:

- Vigorous physical exercise
- Emotional stability
- Intellectual stimulation

Where does it come from?

Dr Kiyo Kitahara developed the approach to work with autistic pupils attending the Musoshino Higashi Kindergarten in Tokyo in 1964 and subsequently opened an elementary school, a junior high school and a high school. The success of the approach with Japanese children, and the international coverage this received, led to the opening in 1987 of the Boston Higashi School. In the late 1980s and early 1990s many UK parents fought to get funding for their child with autism to attend the School in Boston, Massachusetts, and UK children still attend to this day.

Daily Life Therapy is only to be found at the Higashi Schools.

As you will have seen, there are many approaches to education and other complementary therapies that are suitable for children with an ASC. The next step for a parent is the often confusing process of choosing the right school for their child and Polly discusses this in the following chapter.

CHAPTER 8

Choosing a School

A diagnosis of an ASC can complicate the whole concept of education for your child. Clearly, the extent to which this is true will depend on his or her specific needs and abilities, but the very fact that autism has been diagnosed indicates that you will be faced with developmental issues outside the scope of most mainstream educational programmes. Remember to address the health of your child as a priority – no one can learn when they are sick. If your child has abdominal pain or any signs of ill health, this must be addressed first. A healthy child will be able to work to the best of their capacity; a sick child has no chance. Think about when we are sick: we can't do anything – please don't expect your child to be any different.

If your child is two or three and you've only just had a diagnosis, or are awaiting one, you will probably feel that mainstream education is what you will want for your child when the time comes. That's how I felt and I pushed hard for mainstream; for Billy it turned out to be a real mistake. Early intervention programmes often make the world of difference. Remember to look carefully at what is best for your child, though. Getting the wrong programme can set you back, and time means everything with our children. Although many interventions will make a significant difference, you are the parent; never forget that we know our children better than anyone. Instinct is everything.

Whatever happens, the likelihood is that you will have to take more assertive control over your child's education, you may have to try various approaches until you find the right one for you and your child, and you will probably come across more pitfalls than may be the case with children who do not have autism.

Early schooling experiences for Billy

Education for Billy started when he was just over two. Bella was at a wonderful nursery where children just played; there was nothing else but sand pits, dressing-up clothes, toys, painting and singing. My friends' children of a similar age were doing numbers, alphabets and reading books – Bella just played. The head of this nursery was a huge support to me, Billy didn't have a diagnosis at that stage but she could see that I was struggling with him. I was pregnant with Toby, Billy was out of control and Bella had to get to nursery every day. I had no help, so getting a screaming Billy in the car (while heavily pregnant) was a daily battle.

Every day Bella and I drove to the nursery with Billy screaming. The head offered to take Billy for a few mornings a week if I stayed with him. Billy spent his days banging doors and refusing to sit down anywhere. If anyone tried to encourage Billy to 'join in' he would arch his back, scream and attempt to bite or head-butt the person involved. Eventually the head managed to secure funding for Billy to have a one-to-one helper, but it made little difference, as he was so lost in his own world. It was while Billy was attending this nursery that we took part in the *Tonight with Trevor McDonald* programme. What we didn't realise at the time was that this programme would change our lives forever.

When Billy was three I rang a 'very good' local state school to enquire about Bella attending. I spoke to the admissions secretary who was delighted that Bella would be a potential student that September. I then mentioned Billy: 'Also we have a three-year-old that recently has a diagnosis of autism, we would like him to attend your nursery, we would provide the support of course,' I said.

'Oh, I'm sorry Mrs Tommey. We don't take children with special needs like that.'

'Could you at least see him, as he has potential, and with support could do so well in a school like yours,' I pleaded.

'Not possible. We can't take him. We don't do that,' came the brisk reply.

I put the phone down, furious with the school. How dare they not even see Billy? I could accept them turning him down if they at least saw/assessed him, but no, Billy wasn't even worth seeing. 'None of our children will go there,' I told Jon. 'If they won't see Billy then they can't have Bella.'

Jon is, and always has been, the calmer, more pragmatic of the two of us and tried to reason with me, but I was furious, protective and hurt, and nothing was going to make me send my precious children to a school that wouldn't even give Billy a chance. That was the start of a road we hadn't intended to go down: private education.

A change to the private sector

I was in a tricky situation, as our choices were limited. Down the road to us was a large house with a small sign advertising a school, so I made an appointment. The classes were small and the staff friendly. It seemed the perfect transition for Bella. I then mentioned Billy.

The head listened, and then said, 'We would love to take Billy in our nursery. If he needs support then he would have to have that. I can't promise we can meet all his needs, but we will certainly give him a chance.'

So, Bella and Billy started at this school. Both were eligible for nursery vouchers, so paying the fees was manageable. Billy found it hard and so did the school. I remember going to an end of term production that was held in the playground. Each class did a song or dance. Billy's class stood up to stand in a line, and Billy was there! For ten seconds I was so proud. I say ten seconds because that's how long it lasted, he then screamed and ran off, his helper desperately trying to get him back. The more she tried, the louder Billy screamed; he was ruining the song his class were singing. In the end, the helper was told to leave him and the song started again. I sat and watched this class singing while Billy sat on his own running objects repetitively over his eyes, now perfectly happy in his own little world. I would be lying if I didn't tell you how much that hurt. I had ten seconds of complete happiness, then a desperate pain, and a reminder that Billy was so very different from the other children.

Billy's time at this school didn't last long. They tried their best, but they couldn't cope. The final straw was when I got a phone call from the school to say that Billy had been accused of being racist and the parent complaining wanted an explanation immediately. I dashed into school, this was ridiculous, Billy could barely speak and had no interaction with people – how could he be racist? So, there I sat listening to this mother whose young son was in tears because Billy had been running in circles chanting 'whites only, no colours' over and over again. I immediately knew exactly what had happened. Billy was obsessed with our washing machine, the high spin cycle especially. In order to get the high spin noise he loved so much he had to put the machine on – it was on constantly. He had started putting washing in himself, shutting the door and turning it on. Most of our clothes had been wrecked through colours running. When I caught him doing this I would say, 'whites only, no colours' or visa versa. Billy then learned to separate colours so at least our clothes generally stood a better chance. So Billy had been chanting this with his new-found echolaic speech. The mother wasn't convinced. The school tried their best, but it was obvious that this wasn't the right place for Billy.

Our first home programme

It was at this time that we had embarked on a home programme (Lovaas ABA). It was incredibly expensive and involved tutors, head tutors and consultants. To start with Billy did brilliantly, he was taught to sit down on command, pick up various objects and do puzzles. He loved the rewards he got in return and the attention he received for doing so well. The programme started after Billy's health visitor put me in touch with another family with a child who had autism; she thought it would help me realise I was not on my own. I remember the day I first met this family. They were so positive, organised and hopeful that their child would do well, maybe even recover from autism one day.

'Look what he can do,' this mother proudly showed me. 'Thomas, look at me ... touch your nose.' Thomas immediately touched his nose. I was so impressed, I would have given my right arm for Billy to look at me and then on command touch his nose. 'You have to do the Lovaas programme,' she announced.

So that was it. I fought our local education authority and won as many hours as Billy needed to be on this programme.

I have to be honest and say that this was short lived. The problem with Billy and Lovaas, I really believe, is that he couldn't stand the repetitive non-stop demands on him. The final straw for Jon and I came when they were trying to teach Billy to say 'stop it'. Billy was crying, screaming and trying to bite the therapist. I opened the door and found the student therapist pushing Billy, losing her temper. It was unnecessary, to put it mildly, and Billy was starting to lash out on every demand made of him. We stopped the programme and called in the educational department of our LA to help.

Billy had achieved a lot through Lovaas, he had learned to sit down and identify many objects, and his speech was very slowly improving too. That may sound very little to many people but not to us. As the parents who never thought our boy would look at us again, let alone respond to his name, what he had achieved was remarkable. But it had run its course, and he was no longer tolerating it. Many told us to persevere, but I couldn't watch or listen to him screaming for a day longer. I could understand why Billy was so frustrated with it: why, when he knew what an apple was, did he have to be asked over and over again which object an apple was? It was enough to drive anyone mad. That said, many children do really well with Lovaas. As I have said before, not every therapy will suit every person – what works for some may not work for all. So for Billy, yet again, we moved on.

Mainstream school once again, and a new change

The next school was a mainstream state school with a unit attached. I was so excited that my son with autism was going to go to a school with 'typical' children. Someone once told me that if Billy were to mix with 'typical' children then he would stand a good chance of recovery. Now I think differently; for Billy to progress he needs to mix with children and tutors who can encourage him to reach his potential. Our time at this school was also limited. Billy was already aggressive from his final weeks with ABA Lovaas and this school was no better. Billy was expected to sit at a desk and follow instructions, as any other child would do. They even made him sit SATs, in which he got the lowest grade obtainable (mainly because he didn't even sit down; he couldn't – by now he had lost many of the Lovaas skills he had learned). So, Billy started biting anyone and everyone. He pushed a girl over in assembly who was trying to play the violin; he said it was 'bad music'. Eventually a meeting was held and the exclusion officer called. Billy lasted there for just a few terms.

It was becoming clear that, despite our best efforts, Billy's needs were indeed 'special'. We'd looked into all the options in some depth, had tried a variety of mainstream settings with support, we'd tried a home-based ABA approach, and none of it had worked for us. We still had other options to explore and, thankfully, found our way to much more effective support for Billy. As we discovered, what works for one child with autism won't necessarily work for another, and this turns out to be a pretty universal experience. The tricky part is finding your way through to the approach that's right for your child.

Choosing an approach

You may already have an idea of a particular school or programme that you think will meet your child's needs, but do explore all the options and do some research on local schools and services before you decide. Local parents' groups or support groups are bound to include people who are running home programmes, or have tried them, and there's plenty of information on the Net. When it comes to schools, the information provided online from the government has got considerably better in recent years, and you will be able to access a great deal of information on choosing a school, including mainstream and special schools through the Direct Gov website (www.direct.gov.uk/choosingaschool). The links here will help with many aspects of the law, your rights, locating schools, and so on, including plenty of information for special educational needs. Recent government changes may lead to a shake-up of educational bodies and processes in due course. Our advice is to check the website for the Department for Education: www.education.gov.uk.

Home or school?

As we have seen in Chapter 7, some approaches are intrinsic to the school curriculum or used to augment school-based approaches, whereas others are designed to be delivered in the home, either as an 'early intervention' or as an alternative to formal schooling.

A lot will depend on the age of your child, as formal schooling won't kick in until four or five years in most places. The information in the previous chapter on some of the most widely used teaching aids and approaches should be useful as a starting point, and evaluation of these therapies may also be useful to you when it comes to choosing a school.

Early intervention

This essentially means beginning a therapeutic, behavioural or developmental treatment programme with your child prior to formal schooling. This helps to reinforce the neural connections in the brain through its most vigorous stage of development. It establishes learning, communication, sensory integration and motor functioning that may otherwise be missed, especially as autism seems to disrupt or 'short circuit' the natural development of many of these vital connections. There is no doubt at all that the earlier you start to work with your child the better the outcome will be. Remember my advice on health though: no child can do anything if they are in pain. Treat the health issues before even starting to expect your child to learn.

What is the best approach?

There simply is no such thing as 'the best approach'. All of the approaches you hear about (and read about here) have both enthusiastic supporters and outspoken critics, and a lot will depend on your own wishes and philosophies, the specific needs and abilities of your child and how much time, emotional energy, physical energy and (sadly) money you can afford to spend.

When looking at schools and school-based approaches, you will find that many of the specialist schools for children with an ASC are beginning to adopt a combined or holistic approach, incorporating educational programmes with a range of therapeutic approaches and complementary strategies, and it's the overall provision you'll want to see.

Where to begin

Before you decide on the type of approach or combination of approaches you'd like to implement with your child, it is essential to identify the specific issues that have the most impact on his or her behaviour, learning, performance and well-being. Along with the information in this book and elsewhere, this process of evaluation will help you to understand the range or combination of factors that may be contributing to what you might currently see as your child's 'autism features', and should give you vital insight into how best to address them. For example, you might ask yourself:

Does my child

- Appear to be in pain or discomfort?
- Find loud noises or bright lights intolerable?
- Find it difficult to sit still?
- Constantly fidget or 'stim' (see page 172)?
- Reject hugs and cuddles and physical contact?
- Enjoy rough-and-tumble play?
- Get easily distracted?
- Appear to hear but not respond?
- Find it difficult to adapt to new people and situations?
- Avoid eye contact but stare closely at objects?
- Compulsively touch objects or surfaces?
- Shout and make loud or shrill noises?
- Have constant diarrhoea or constipation?
- Walk on tiptoes?
- Have difficulty organising or sequencing tasks?
- Adopt strange postures or rub up against the furniture?
- Reject certain foodstuffs and demand others?
- Have red ears or dark circles around the eyes?

This is not a comprehensive list, and it's probably more helpful to compile your own based on your own unique knowledge of your child, but many items on this generic list of typical characteristics can result from issues that are separate and distinct from the core deficits of autism (the triad of impairments doesn't mention hyper- or hyposensitivities or gastrointestinal issues), and may be directly helped through nutritional interventions or educational and therapeutic approaches. Whatever the specific combination of issues that affect your child, these must be uppermost in your mind when deciding on the best approach for you.

Statement of Special Educational Needs (SEN)

If your child is in an early education setting or in school and either you or they feel that he or she is having difficulties, needs lots of extra help or is not making enough progress, then they might start to make extra provision (more help, special equipment, and so on) through something called 'early years action' or 'school action'.

If this is insufficient to meet your child's needs, then either you or the school can ask the LA to carry out a statutory assessment. If your child has a diagnosis of an ASC, this is quite likely to happen, but will depend on his or her particular needs. If your child clearly needs specialist help right from the start, then you'll probably already be in touch with the relevant professionals, and this process will kick in virtually automatically.

The statutory assessment or 'statementing' process is governed by the SEN Code of Practice, which gives formal guidance to LAs on how to consult with parents and conduct the necessary assessments within a statutory framework (including a timeline, which will be no longer than six months). The outcome of statutory assessment is likely to be the production of a Statement of Special Educational Needs (known as a Statement), which contains details about your child's needs and how they might best be met. The LA has to consult with you on their proposals before they finalise the Statement, and the final step is the decision about the most appropriate school or other education provision.

The Statement is essentially a legally binding commitment by the LA to provide the services that your child needs, based on their assessment, so you'll need the Statement to access special education unless you can afford to go private.

At the time of going to press, this information is correct but due to a current review of services by the Coalition government, some aspects may change. Regularly updated information on developments in SEN is available at www.education.gov.uk and www.teachernet.gov.uk.

Choosing a school

When it comes to choosing a school for your child with an ASC you will already be aware of many of the factors that you will need to take into account. You may already have formulated some idea of the type of education provision you would prefer, or the type of help you think your child needs; perhaps informed by the outcomes of any interventions and strategies you may have already tried, heard about, researched or had recommended to you. Don't feel at all bad if you're still fully stuck in the 'I just don't know' zone – most of us spend a lot of time there. It's a steep and tricky learning curve and far from an exact science. Every child is different and may or may not respond well to different types of provision, intervention or approach.

Even if you are contemplating starting or continuing a home-based programme once your child reaches school age, it's wise to explore the options, and there are, of course, many variables.

For many of you, the overwhelming priority will be to find a school within reasonable striking distance that will meet your child's needs in accordance with your wishes and/or expectations, and which meets the criteria for funding within your LA. The processes involved are complex, as you might imagine, but the following sections might be of help to you at various stages.

Types of school

There are many different types of school, but at the point of choosing, the most important things to consider are to do with the specific provision (whether you opt for a mainstream or special school and what curriculum/programmes/specialist support, and so on, they actually offer), the skills and training of the staff, and the funding arrangements; that is, will the LA pay for your child to attend? These are, of course, highly complex questions, and there are too many variables for us to be able to do them justice here; however, it's worth knowing that you have certain legal rights and, in the UK, the LA has certain legal duties and responsibilities. The different categories of schools are listed overleaf.

Categories of schools in the UK

Main categories	Owned and/or run by
Community schools	LA
Foundation schools and trust schools	Governing body or charitable foundation
Voluntary-aided schools	Governing body or charitable foundation
Voluntary-controlled schools	LA

Types of school in the UK and their characteristics

Types of school	Characteristics
Specialist schools	(The majority of secondary schools and all academies.) Follow the National Curriculum, but specialise in a particular subject or curriculum area, such as sport, visual arts, science or technology.
Academies	Publicly funded independent schools, often set up with the support of charitable or corporate sponsors. Free from local government control and they have a flexible curriculum with specialist status
City technical colleges	Independent but non fee-paying, emphasis on science, technology and vocational qualifications

Types of school	Characteristics
Community and foundation special schools (maintained special schools)	For children with physical or learning difficulties (with SEN Statement) whose needs cannot be met in mainstream education
Non-maintained special schools	Often highly specialised special schools. Owned by charitable trusts, run by a governing body. Fee-paying but not for profit. Fees are usually paid by LA
Faith schools	Run like most state schools but may have admissions criteria and curriculum reflecting the particular faith group
Grammar schools	Select all or most pupils based on academic ability
Maintained boarding schools	No fees for tuition, but charges for boarding
Residential special schools	Many special schools for people with an ASC have a residential component. Education and residential care is usually joint-funded between LA education and social services departments
Independent schools	Funded through fees from parents and financial investment. Most have charitable status
Independent special schools	Schools run by charities or charitable trusts for children with SEN statements, often for those with the most complex and severe needs. Fees may be paid privately or by LA

Rights and responsibilities

You are entitled to at least 15 hours per week of free nursery, playgroup or preschool provision from either the September or the January following your child's third birthday (depending on the date of birth) right up until compulsory school age (the term following the fifth birthday). You may also be eligible for help with the cost of additional childcare. Types and standards will, of course, differ and you might not be able to get your first choice, but you have a right to something.

When it comes to choosing a school, your rights in law will depend on the provisions detailed in the Statement, so don't agree the proposed Statement until you're sure it accurately describes your child's needs and offers suitable support – and don't agree a school until you've explored all the options.

The default position is that your child should be educated in a mainstream school unless:

- This would not meet your child's needs, or would adversely affect the education of the other children, and no reasonable adjustments to the organisation of the school could make it work.

- You opt for a special school. You have a right to express a preference, and the LA must consider it, but you will need a Statement, and will need to be able to demonstrate that your child's needs cannot be met in a mainstream setting.

- You decide to educate your child at home (defined as 'education otherwise').

If the LA suggests a special school, you still have the right to choose a mainstream school, but the LA doesn't have a duty to provide it if they can demonstrate that such a placement would be to the detriment of the efficient education of the other pupils. They would also have to demonstrate that no reasonable adjustments would make such a placement work. You do not have an absolute right to either a special or a mainstream place.

In among all this is the duty of the LA to spend their budget efficiently, so money definitely comes into it, as they have to balance finite resources across the needs of all the children in their area. However, if you're not happy with their decision or think that they're underestimating your child's additional needs, you need to make your concerns clear to the authority. This would be via the Special Educational Needs and Disability (SEND) tribunal.

The right school for your child

There are far too many variables for us to go into in detail here, as the factors that you will consider in coming to your decision about what type of schooling to go for will be unique to you, your child and your wishes. What we can do, however, is set out some pointers that may be helpful to you.

- You do not have to do this alone, so seek advice and support. Every LA has a duty to provide help and support to parents of children with SEN.
- When arranging to meet with LA teams or officers, be prepared to make appointments several weeks in advance.
- Make yourself known to Social Services. You might not feel you need Social Service support at the moment, but the SEN team within your local Social Services department can arrange helpful support, such as occupational therapy assessment and respite breaks. It makes sense to look into the support available sooner rather than later.

Mainstream or special?

In the first instance, this might seem like an easy one, and you may be guided by your own existing opinions about the best way to educate your child. Of course, as with every element of this process, everything depends on the specific issues affecting your child. Some children with an ASC, like Billy, are unable to cope with the academic demands of a mainstream curriculum, and may also not cope with or benefit from the social elements or the 'hidden' curriculum that happens within and between lessons, or in the playground or cafeteria, and so on, and may find the general hubbub of a mainstream setting distracting and confusing. Remember how excited I was that Billy was going to a 'normal, typical' school? This turned out to be the worst decision for Billy. It's hard, but you have to think of what is best for your child rather than what will make you as a parent feel better.

The other side of this is that, while a special school is likely to be organised specifically for the needs of children like your own, you might feel that they may lose out on the potential benefits of 'peer-assisted' learning, a more academic curriculum, or the normalising influence of a mainstream classroom, as their peers will have much the same types of need and ability as themselves.

It is helpful to consider carefully whether your child has the skills and abilities that are necessary to be able to access aspects such as peer-assisted learning, role-modelling, active learning in groups, and so on. If not, then a mainstream setting could be counterproductive, or you may find yourselves having to fight for more and more additional support and special arrangements to enable your child to access the curriculum. I have spoken to many parents who say that while their child has coped with the academics in a mainstream setting they have struggled terribly with the social aspect of this. One mother told me that her son literally had no friends.

If you lean towards inclusion in a mainstream setting, you will clearly want to know the specific types of provision and additional support that are available in your local mainstream schools, and particularly what they offer by way of specialist training and experience supporting children with autism.

- Think about the reality your child faces: what they find hard to do and what they will struggle to achieve. In other words, what do they need now and what type of setting is best placed to teach those skills? Consider his or her potential, interests, personality, and so on.

- What are your dreams and fears? Do they make sense in the context of your understanding of autism? Academic learning may be accessible to your child intellectually, but looking to the future, applying this to a fruitful working life and a measure of true independence may be an entirely different issue.

- Take some time to discuss as a family what your hopes, wishes, fears and aspirations are. Draw up a list that covers those elements that you feel to be essential in any school you choose and those that you feel to be desirable. Make sure to include any things that you might consider 'deal breakers' one way or the other; for example, single sex, distance from home, facilities, class sizes, pupil–staff ratios, experience and expertise, staff training, and specific educational or therapeutic approaches.

- Think about several options, including a change of school at junior or secondary age. What you decide now does not necessarily dictate your child's entire school life, and (for example) early intervention and special schooling in the infant and primary phases may make a difference to your options at secondary transfer.

- Conversely, if you decide that mainstream schooling is your desired option in primary education, you may still find that secondary schooling is an entirely different prospect. Primary education is typically a more controllable teaching and learning environment both academically and socially, whereas secondary education is much more reliant on independence, social maturity and self-motivation – and it demands a whole new skill set.

- If you decide on special schooling, you might still want to consider whether you would want an ASC specialist school or whether a more generic special school might offer some of the benefits of special education while retaining some of the more social and/or academic benefits of mainstream.

- Start to make a record of your ideas, as you might need to refer back in order to remind yourself about the pros and cons of each option.

Day or residential?

Again, this may seem simple according to your wishes, and of course will depend on the age and specific needs of your child, but you might want to consider the pros and cons of a residential placement if that's something that seems accessible (if it's something that could be offered through a joint-funding arrangement between your LA Education and Social Services departments, for instance).

Although you may instinctively feel that your child should be within the family for all the social benefits this confers, you may again wish to consider whether these potential benefits are actually accessible to him at the moment.

A residential placement may be offered if your child's behavioural and/or independence needs are such that 24-hour education, care and behavioural support are required, or if your own situation is such that you cannot cope with these demands. The fact that you, as parents, also need care and support from your LA may also be a factor in this.

It may be the case that you feel that a '24-hour curriculum' would be of significant benefit to your child and his or her development, in which case it may be worth your while to seek a specialist placement that offers this. Of course, funding arrangements are critical within LAs, and it is unlikely that you will receive funding for such a placement unless your child's needs (and/or your needs) truly demand it; however, the social and life-skills elements of a curriculum for people with an ASC are widely recognised as crucial to their overall development, and (from the LA's point of view) can be of such benefit that they save true-life costs further down the line for all concerned in terms of health, well-being, social support, mental health and income support.

Another consideration may be that the provision you consider to be appropriate to meet your child's needs may be some way from your home, so you might need to balance the pros of family life with the cons of daily travel.

Gather information

Look into both mainstream and special schools – and even residential provision. Try to keep an open mind until you weigh it all up to make your decision. Try to balance all the pros and cons and gather as much information as possible about the available options.

- Collect brochures from as many schools as possible, and then try to match what they offer with what you are looking for.

- Do your own research online; most schools these days have their own websites and you can start to get a feel for a school by (for instance) how up-to-date the information is and how prominent their information is about special needs or ASCs, or any element in which you are particularly interested, as this shows how prominent they want to make it. All current and relatively recent Ofsted reports are available online at www.ofsted.gov.uk.

- Look at both LA schools and independent schools, and apply your list of desirables and essentials to them. Always send for a copy of the school magazine or brochure. This may be available as a download from the website – or just phone the school.

- If you are interested in particular schools, read their Ofsted reports and look at the school's Web page. Is it current? Does the information match the findings of the Ofsted report? Ofsted reports are not a particularly accurate gauge of what a school can offer, but they do look in some detail at behaviour support, educational outcomes, teaching and learning, special needs, specialist interventions, social and pastoral support, management and training – all the things that you'd want to look into yourself. They can certainly help and may furnish you with specific questions to ask if you go on a visit.

- If you want to ask any questions, or arrange a visit, phone the school and make an appointment. Don't be put off if the head is busy; heads are busy, and the deputy, or assistant head, or the SENCO (special educational needs coordinator) or admissions officer (depending on the school) will be able to give you the information you need.

- Some schools only offer group open days. That's OK, as it will give you a chance to look around without the pressure of a face-to-face meeting with a senior manager. It may be the case that all you get from this is generic information about the school, but it should be enough to give you a feel for the place, and, if you're interested in a place, you should then arrange a personal interview, furnished with pertinent and specific questions.

School visits

Go prepared to make notes, and if you find you have questions or concerns as you walk around, raise them, or note them down for your next visit.

- You can tell a lot about the culture of a school by how they welcome and treat visitors. You should expect to be warmly greeted and made to feel welcome. In a school where the staff are happy and well managed you can expect to be smiled at or greeted by staff and pupils as you move through the school. If a member of staff asks if they can help you, or asks who you are, this is a sign that they are professional and vigilant. Don't take this as an absolute, as staff should also be busy, on-task and may be otherwise occupied, but your reception is important to the feeling that you're left with.

- Look at displays. Are they current? Would they make sense to your child? If this is a special school, the way that information is conveyed through displays, signs and symbols is of vital importance. Verbal skills, literacy skills and symbol use should be central to the curriculum offering and you should be able to see the considered work and expertise of the staff in how they present information.

In communal or staff areas, read notices intended for both staff and pupils. What can you detect from the information and the tone of it?

- Listen to the noise/sound level in school, playground and dining hall. Would this be an issue for your child?

- Listen to what the teachers and support staff are saying to the children. Is language-use measured and structured? All children with an ASC, even in the high-functioning range, and even in a mainstream environment, will need spoken language to be limited and structured to aid understanding and to avoid confusion.

- If you witness behavioural problems or even physical management of pupils by staff, don't jump to conclusions. Put your observations in the context of your own child's needs. Observe how the staff respond. Does there appear to be a system in operation? Is the response calm and measured? You can ask your tour guide for an explanation of what happened and how the school's policies were enacted, or save it up to ask the head or another senior person later. You might also take the opportunity to ask how the school would deal with any particular behavioural issues that affect your own child.

- Make sure you get to see any special facilities, therapies or programmes that interest you. Having a resource in a school is not the same as using it effectively. For instance, a multi-sensory room is an expensive and attractive resource, but you might want to ask how often it's accessed by children and how often the therapist visits.

- If you're able to observe lunchtime (or any meal), see if the school capitalises on the powerful and multiple opportunities for functional communication and life-skills learning that this affords. Do the teachers or support staff eat with the pupils? Is it clear that learning programmes are incorporated into mealtime? Is the food on offer appropriate: healthy, balanced and versatile to particular dietary requirements?

- If toileting and continence issues are a factor for you, you'll want to find out whether the school can provide support for children who are in nappies, not fully continent or toilet trained.

- If this seems like a positive school, you can write to the headteacher requesting an interview, with a list of questions arising from your preliminary visit. The head may respond in writing to your queries, or will be ready with answers when you meet.

Curriculum

You can ask for copies of the school's policies on any issue, so if you'd like to see their policy on teaching and learning, behaviour support, child protection, physical management, language and communication, then ask.

- The staff training policy is key to how seriously the school takes its responsibilities to ensure that members of staff are equipped with current understanding and strategies.

- Curriculum policies should describe how individual subjects or learning areas are taught, along with information on the resources available.

- You can ask to see a lesson in progress in order to observe teaching methods, although the school is perfectly at liberty to say no. Some schools prefer not to take visitors into classes due to the disruption this may cause, and this is to be respected. But you can ask about all these issues.

- Whether this is a mainstream or special school, their understanding of the particular needs of children with autism is paramount for your child. You could ask whether any members of staff have specific autism qualifications and experience, and in a specialist school, you would expect there to be plenty.

- Ask what the school considers itself to specialise in with regard to its pupils (particularly those with special needs or an ASC). Is it learning, social skills, behaviour, vocational education, and so on? What does it excel in?

- In a mainstream setting, find out what specific strategies the school employs to ensure access to the curriculum for children with an ASC, and how they manage anxiety.

- Anxiety is an issue for children with an ASC in any setting. Does the school use specific strategies such as relaxation, breathing techniques or massage?

- How does the school manage pupil motivation and reward performance? Do they operate a reward system and/or a series of sanctions? Are children rewarded for their achievements?

- How does the school adapt the National Curriculum (NC) to make sense to a child with an ASC? There is a lot more freedom these days as to how schools can interpret the NC. You'll clearly want to see how they do this; for example, do they offer a limited curriculum, or take longer over key stages? Do they offer vocational qualifications such as NVQ or ASDAN? How do they record progress?

- Ask to look at a sample IEP (individual education programme). The IEP is what schools have to produce (according to the SEN Code of Practice) to plan and demonstrate what special targets or teaching and learning strategies they will employ in order to meet a child's needs as set out in the SEN Statement. This should show you how much effort the school puts into their additional responsibilities to pupils with a statement or, in the case of a special school, how they arrange individual learning programmes to meet individual needs. Targets should be clear enough to show you exactly what the school plans for the pupil to learn over a given period on top of the overall curriculum offering.

- Ask for an overview of the school year so that you can see what plans they have made for outings, special projects, trips, adventures, and so on.

- Through all of this, your overriding concern must be whether this environment and these approaches will meet the needs of your child. Will he or she be motivated, well managed and treated with care and respect, will they get the support they need and will they learn?

- Ask about home–school communication. You will want to feel that the school considers you a partner in the education and care of your child, so it is important to consider the extent and nature of information the school provides. How often can you expect updates? How regularly are parents invited to the school to view work, talk to staff, and so on? Are parents invited to attend training courses and participate in school activities? Is there a 'home–school diary' or some way of maintaining an ongoing dialogue between you and the school?

- If you can talk to other parents, or to the parent governor (every school has at least one, depending on its size), you'll get a good idea of the role of parents in the school and the quality of the information provided by the school.

Specialist therapies and interventions

Access to, and support from, individual therapists may be something that the school is able to offer itself. Some schools, particularly non-maintained and independent special schools, employ therapists such as speech and language therapists (SALT), occupational therapists (OT) and massage therapists; however, it is still more usual for such specialists, especially SALTs and OTs, to be employed by the NHS and allocated time with individual children through the provisions listed in their individual SEN Statements.

Although many children receive individual therapy, these days the SALT is much more likely to work in the classroom (especially in primary and special schools) working with groups, supporting individuals, advising and collaborating with teachers and classroom assistants on strategies to improve functional language and communication skills across the curriculum.

If your child's Statement details speech and language therapy and/or occupational therapy provision (it would be highly unusual for a Statement for a child with an ASC diagnosis not to specify speech and language therapy provision), it's worthwhile looking into how this will be provided. How often is the therapist in school? How is time allocated? Are children withdrawn for individual sessions or is it classroom-based? How are achievement targets drawn up? Is the therapist employed by the school or by the NHS? This could make a difference as to how the therapist works, as it may mean that she or he is not necessarily subject to the school's own policies and approaches.

If you get a chance to talk to the SALT and/or OT directly (you could request this when you make your appointment), ask them about how they work with children and how they collaborate with the school to meet its aims.

If your child is on a specialist diet or takes dietary supplements, or you think these approaches might be necessary, ask whether the school will support this; that is, do they cater for specialist diets (such as a GFCF diet) through their own kitchen or catering supplier, or would this have to be provided through a packed lunch? Would they be prepared to give dietary supplements you provide (such as digestive dietary enzymes prior to lunch)?

If dietary and nutritional factors are a key issue for you, as they are for us, then these are important questions.

Happiness

Taking into account all the ins and outs of provision, education and therapy, the school environment, staff and resources, the decision about which school would be best for your child can effectively be condensed into what will make you and your child happy.

Follow your instincts. The 'feel' you get for a school is an important factor in how comfortable you will be for your child to spend the majority of his or her waking life there for the next few years. Take in as much as possible, and believe the evidence of your own eyes and ears rather than any preconceptions, recommendations or hype. Trust yourself as the parent: you know your child better than anyone.

Remember that the people you meet on a visit may become vital and regular fixtures in your life for a while, so imagine yourself building relationships with them. It can only be a rough guide, especially on a brief visit, but if the staff seem happy, the school is likely to be a happy place.

Imagine your child there. What will he or she like about it and what might become an issue? You'll want your child to learn and develop, and to achieve this they will have to be challenged and stretched, but you'll also want them to be happy, and to want to go every day.

Billy is now at an excellent school; he is a weekly boarder and loves it. Billy is happy because he has the right people around him, and he is taught life skills as well as classroom work. The staff have the right attitude with Billy – he knows his boundaries, and therefore he can cope. The school works on the method that each individual is unique and has their own programme designed for them. The children work in groups with a tutor. They do a lot of exercise and the school caters for the many different diets that the children require. Billy became a weekly residential student at 13, it was a very difficult day when we made that decision, but one that now we are glad we made. Billy is incredibly happy, it took some time to get this right, but now we are here it makes every bit of difference to have a happy child. If you had asked me a year previously if I would let Billy go to a residential setting I would have been horrified. But, we knew Billy would be happy there and he is and, most importantly, he is progressing on a weekly basis. Finding the right environment is crucial – it may take some time as it did for Billy, but it makes all the difference when you get there.

In Part 3 we detail the range of options for learning and nutrition that we have discovered through living with Billy and which we believe help to improve the lives of children with autism. I begin with the combination of learning approaches, called Whole Health Learning.

PART 3

THE WAY FORWARD: WHOLE HEALTH LEARNING AND NUTRITION

CHAPTER 9

Whole Health Learning

Our experience in living and working with Billy, combined with his most successful school experience and the knowledge (and knowledgeable people) we've picked up along the way, have taught us a great deal about the range of options available to help improve the lives of those with autism. Over the last few years it has become increasingly clear to us that, aside from the stories we all hear about miraculous recoveries attributable to one type of intervention, there are a number of common threads running through many success stories. Our conclusion is that improving the lives of our children depends on finding a combination of approaches that meets all their needs. It seems increasingly likely that the way autism manifests in different children is due to a whole range of different causal and contributory factors, so it stands to reason that it will take a similar range of interventions and approaches to address it. This may seem like an obvious conclusion, but the difference is that no organisation at the moment is offering such a range of strategies and, until now, finding anything like this has been a frustrating process of trial and error for parents.

Our thoughts on this came together while planning our 2009 Autism Trust conference to bring together the best minds and most effective approaches from across the educational, therapeutic and biomedical fields, and through our quest to weave the best and most effective ideas together to support Billy and people like him through schooldays and into adulthood. Because our approach is holistic and eclectic, we have called it Whole Health Learning.

In describing Whole Health Learning, we have not focused on any specifics of 'the curriculum' (that is, specific educational programmes or academic learning or qualifications), because we see this approach as being applicable to a range of different types of schools and adult provision that can be combined with other approaches; however, our ideal involves the vocational curriculum approach that has been so successful for Billy. Some aspects of this approach are already available in certain schools, and we will be campaigning hard to introduce it to others and to train practitioners in the necessary disciplines – it is also central to our plans for the Autism Trust's Centres of Excellence. In the meantime, the individual components of Whole Health Learning are strategies that we believe every person with autism should have access to and that you might want to seek out.

What is Whole Health Learning?

Whole Health Learning is a holistic approach to the education and personal development of children and adults with an ASC. It has been developed by The Autism Trust to incorporate the best practice and most effective strategies we've come across to address all aspects of the physical and emotional health and well-being of those with an ASC. It recognises that all the elements that make up an individual's nature, health, constitution and learning ability are interrelated and must all be acknowledged, accommodated and supported for learning to take place.

This approach demands specific attention to the whole-health needs of each individual and it encompasses:

- Physical fitness
- Good health (wellness)
- Calmness

- Self-esteem and self-efficacy
- Emotional well-being
- Personal development
- Social development
- Independence

Whole Health Learning comprises a range of specific, person-centred strategies that seek to address difficulties and vulnerabilities in all these areas, thereby promoting the development of healthy and independent adults with a range of relevant skills. These strategies include:

- Structured environments
- Biomedical treatments where necessary
- Developmental movement
- Graphic support
- Massage and aromatherapy
- Diet, nutrition and hydration
- Exercise and relaxation
- Social, play and leisure activities

How Billy's learning developed

After a few disasters and false starts, Billy's education started to come together, and the years of his educational life from age 7 until 14 have been considerably more successful. In this chapter, we will tell you what it was that worked so well and introduce you to our considered opinion of the most effective combination of approaches. In doing so, we will bring together many of the issues we've covered in this book.

We have said before that every child is different, and we stand by that wholeheartedly, but there are clearly many common strands, and it is through finding versatile, creative and adaptive ways to deal specifically with these common issues that many of you may find the progress and peace of mind you seek.

When Billy was seven he started at a specialist school for children with autism and Asperger's syndrome. Of course it took a little while to settle, especially as he'd been out of school and at home with us for so long, but these people knew what they were doing. They knew exactly who and what they were taking on and, before long, things started to change for the better. For one thing, Billy was happy to go to school every day!

Meeting the principal, Stephanie Lord, was a revelation and a significant turning point in our lives, as here was someone (finally) who truly understood the whole range of issues that affect children like Billy. Stephanie had developed an approach through years of experience that was not only finely tuned to these issues but was also bold, creative and far sighted.

Stephanie is a leader in her field. She has been headteacher of three schools for children with an ASC and has consistently pushed the boundaries of education and expectation for people with autism through her energy, creativity and commitment as well as through her intuitive understanding of the holistic, whole-health needs of people on the spectrum. Stephanie was promoting calming strategies, massage, aromatherapy, physical fitness, diet, hydration, structured language, visual environments and sensory-motor activities as essential components of ASC education many years before the rest of the world started to catch up and 'well-being' became a buzz word in education.

When Billy started at his new school, like so many children who enter special education having failed to thrive in mainstream, he had very few age-appropriate skills, very limited language, no literacy or numeracy skills to speak of and few of the strategies that we now know can help and support children with an ASC. Consequently he didn't really know how to 'be' in a school environment, as his experience was that school made no sense. Any skills that he may have learned through ABA (see page 144) were not generalised outside the ABA setting and, although he was generally passive and smiley, and tolerated the presence of others (adults and other children), he showed little awareness of what the others were for. He was anxious and unwilling to work in a group and was prone to bouts of crying and occasional aggressive outbursts. He had poor body awareness, low self-esteem, tight muscles and posture, limited physical and cognitive flexibility and little stamina for work. He had no real awareness of routine, where he was in his day, what he was able or unable to do, and no structured ways of seeking help.

Thankfully, Stephanie and her staff were excellent at addressing precisely these kinds of issues. The whole culture of the school viewed learning not as an isolated set of skills and behaviours to be ticked off one at a time, but as a holistic process that must acknowledge and accommodate all aspects of autism at all times. The staff understood that many of the behavioural elements of autism, including stereotyped or 'challenging' behaviour, are outcomes of anxiety and discomfort arising from individual social, perceptual and physical circumstances. They understood the devastating effect on children with ASCs of their disordered social and sensory perceptions and thought processes, and organised the curriculum around a range of measures to promote calm and well-being and to instil a structured understanding of the rules, responsibilities and wider implications of real-life and social interactions. Moreover, they did this in a way that was focused on students learning to manage their own calming, physical well-being, communication and coping strategies.

Social skills open doors to the future

Perhaps most significantly in terms of preparing children with ASCs for independent life, the school understood that however accessible academic learning may seem to be for people with an ASC, particularly those with high-functioning autism and Asperger's syndrome, the reality was rather different. The profound deficits in social communication, social interaction and imaginative thought processes inherent in the diagnosis of autism often render socially detached academic study futile, and even counterproductive, in the real world of work and adult life, and so outweigh this when it comes to prioritising learning and development. There are too many adults with ASCs out there already with academic qualifications but no jobs, because they have never learned the skills necessary to manage a working life or conduct themselves in the workplace. Consequently, the focus of the school was on teaching fundamental work and life skills, including strategies for thinking, planning, communicating and managing their interactions and anxieties, rather than pursuing academic study for its own sake.

The academic content of the school curriculum was therefore embedded in vocational activities and in the day-to-day life of the centre, which also had a residential department and a flourishing training and professional-development department. Students' daily lives revolved around their involvement in the running of the school and centre, including horticulture and site maintenance around the extensive gardens and grounds; cleaning and servicing the many school and centre buildings; catering and hospitality for staff, students, visitors and course delegates; and various administrative, business and reception duties. All the children were involved in this 'live' work at various levels, culminating at the upper end of the school in vocational qualifications (NVQ) in these areas, but starting with a range of routine tasks and jobs woven in and around physical, therapeutic, creative and educational activities. Reading, writing, verbal communication, science, maths and many other aspects of the National Curriculum were delivered as intrinsic, functional elements of daily work, daily life and self-organisation, rather than as discrete subjects.

In Billy's class, as well as these structured 'jobs', he was also taught fundamental developmental skills to help him to 'be' in class. Simple things like greeting, sitting, looking, waiting in line, turn-taking, asking for help, moving around the school, and so on, were all explicitly taught and supported by graphics, a structured environment and structured language.

Connected learning

The school taught children the connections between the various aspects of their daily lives and showed them elements of 'the big picture' that would otherwise be inaccessible to them and may be the source of much confusion and anxiety. This 'connected learning' approach makes explicit (through structured language, structured teaching and graphic representation) the rules that govern conduct and communication in various places and situations: the thought processes involved in planning and organising; the differences between formal and informal, private and public, work and leisure; the reasons why things happen or are done a certain way; the motivations, expectations and reactions of others; the way the body reacts to stress and anxiety, and how to bring it all under conscious control.

The connected learning ethos focuses on five strands of thinking and learning that help children develop strategies to understand and manage their own anxiety and physical responses, their own work and organisation, their interactions with other people, and their awareness of their own role in events; it is called BERIS: Body basics, Environment, Relatedness, Insight and Self-belief. These five BERIS strands also provide staff with a structured 'way of seeing' the needs and actions of the pupils for the purposes of planning and offering support.

Body basics – we learn to be calm

Understanding body basics helps to connect children to what their own body is doing. It helps them read the bodily signs of stress, such as an increased heart rate and breathing rate, and to apply specific coping strategies and support structures; for example: I put my hand on my head to think, I put my hand on my chest to breathe. I can breathe and blow; I can have time alone; I can ask for a massage.

Environment – we learn to use systems of work

A range of structures is utilised to help children connect to organised thinking, motivation and planning, including extensive graphical support strategies, enabling them to access support materials matching their own learning style and without complex spoken instructions. These include individualised personal organisers, timetables, work schedules, mind-maps, task instructions and rules.

Relatedness – we learn to relate and interact

Understanding the roles and actions of others in the environment is clearly one of the key issues in autism. This strand uses a range of approaches, particularly graphics and structured and standardised forms of words – or 'mantras' – to help children connect people with their roles in an interaction and to clarify expectations and boundaries, making explicit what would otherwise be implicit and inaccessible; for example, 'your task is … ', 'the rule is …', 'I am waiting for you to …'

Insight – we learn to think about what we do

In this context, insight is about reflection and problem-solving, helping children to make connections between actions and their consequences and between strategies and outcomes. Insight focuses on supporting children to reflect on why things happen, what went wrong and what went right, what they find hard and what they find easy in a given situation and on selecting strategies that can help, including using an organiser, calming techniques, mantras and social stories (see page 163).

Self-belief – we learn that we have responsibilities and rights

Issues of poor self-esteem and low self-confidence are often debilitating for people with autism, as much of their experience is negative: 'getting things wrong' or that they 'can't do it'. Finding internal appreciation of success for its own sake, and appreciation of the implicit approval of others as a social reward are inaccessibly complex social constructs for people with an ASC. Self-belief, however, connects the other strands of BERIS as a tool-kit for success, making success and approval explicit through positive praise and rewards, and it supports children to recognise their own options and abilities.

Changes for Billy

Billy soon began to thrive within this highly structured learning environment. His ability to be with others improved, he began to see the adults in school as sources of help and reassurance, and could take himself to a calm place if things got too much for him – furthermore, his episodes of crying and biting were significantly reduced. He began to imitate others in shared play, enjoyed movement games, running and cycling activities with the group, and his reading, writing and counting improved – particularly when counting the points he had earned towards a reward – and he started to show his talents on the computer!

Billy was happy and settled for years, and had made tremendous progress, but sadly all good things must come to an end, and unfortunately the school changed beyond recognition following a reorganisation of management and direction. Eventually, when Billy was 13 it came time for him to move on, and we made the extraordinarily difficult decision to opt for a residential placement at a newly opened school that promised the same ethos and the same combination of approaches that we had had so much success with before.

We count ourselves extremely fortunate that our first forays into special schooling were so successful and that Billy was once again settled and happy in his new school and is progressing in leaps and bounds. Not only has it helped Billy and us towards a more optimistic future but it has also helped to shape our ideas about the kind of approaches that other children like Billy can benefit from and that will continue to support Billy as he becomes an adult.

What is involved in Whole Health Learning?

Here is a brief overview of the approaches that are integral to Whole Health Learning:

Structured environments

Nothing should be left to chance in the active support of people with an ASC. Every consideration should be given to the specific impairments inherent in the condition, and these will include the organisation of the physical environment, the presentation of materials, the measured use of language and personal interventions, the organisation of graphic support materials and the need for person-centred approaches.

Biomedical treatments

Many people with an ASC suffer from a variety of treatable biomedical conditions, such as vitamin and mineral deficiencies, metabolic imbalances, food and chemical intolerances and gastrointestinal conditions, which may be responsible for many behavioural and developmental symptoms. Biomedical treatment protocols, involving nutritional supplements, enriched diets and exclusion diets, can have a dramatic effect on many autistic symptoms and may address some of the underlying causes.

Developmental movement

People with an ASC will have difficulties with sensory perception issues, communication skills and forming personal relationships, which are partly caused by missing links in the early development of the brain. Developmental movement programmes incorporate activities which are designed to address these issues by bridging fundamental gaps in physical and emotional development and breaking down the sensitivities that have arisen through impaired sensory integration.

Graphic support

The key problems for people with an ASC are the difficulties that they experience when communicating socially, especially when holding conversations and thinking imaginatively. People who have difficulties in these areas experience high levels of anxiety and, consequently, behavioural issues. Ways to help are by representing language concepts, social narratives, ideas and thought processes visually. This is achieved by using graphics: written text, symbols and photographs.

Massage and aromatherapy

Partly caused by sensory integration difficulties in early childhood development, many people with an ASC are resistant to touch that is nurturing and they therefore miss out on how it can benefit their overall development. Massage and aromatherapy programmes have a proven record in breaking down issues of tactile defensiveness, bringing specific health and well-being benefits by reducing stress and anxiety, and by promoting relaxation, self-awareness, improved body-image and physical revitalisation.

Diet, nutrition and hydration

An essential part of Whole Health Learning focuses on diet, nutrition and hydration, and this will be discussed fully in Chapter 10.

Exercise and relaxation

Physical exercise has phenomenal health benefits, and proper relaxation is essential for the maintenance of the body's equilibrium and for managing stress.

All people should do at least 30 minutes of moderate physical exercise at least five times a week, but most people do too little.

Whole Health Learning promotes both exercise and relaxation for the physical and psychological well-being of people with an ASC.

Social, play and leisure activities

Although social, play and leisure activities are meant to be fun, they are also instrumental in teaching children fundamental lessons about how the world works. In adulthood, imaginative play translates as fantasising or creative thinking, but adults also play – that is, they engage in activities just for fun or for the social benefits. People with autism are known to have specific problems with imaginative play, but it's never too late to use fun and creative activities to rehearse real-life situations and to gain the well-being benefits of relaxed enjoyment of life.

The effects of stress

Stress is also a common feature of ASCs and can affect a person mentally, physically and emotionally. Stress can upset the body's blood sugar levels, as well as reducing the effectiveness of the digestive system, promoting heightened sensitivities, increasing irritability and an inability to concentrate, as well as creating obsessive thinking, chronic tension and anxiety; it can also cause chronic depression or boredom and aggressive outbursts.

We respond to stress physically through sweating, an increased heart rate and breathing rate, as well as headaches, backaches, tight muscles and changes in appetite, or even nausea. As well as using stress management techniques, there are a number of nutritional therapies that can be applied to support the function of the adrenal glands. The role of the adrenal glands is to respond to stressful situations, by releasing hormones that control the stress response. Commonly, the adrenal glands in people with autism are depleted and therefore need nutritional support; otherwise they can interact with the thyroid and thymus glands thereby reducing the body's immune defences against pathogens.

Finding the way forward

The most important thing here is that you do the right thing for your child – but knowing what that is will be the problem. A school that embraces the Whole Health Learning principles will look at your child as an individual and advise you on the best way that they can move forward, develop and grow.

Billy came on leaps and bounds with Whole Health Learning, mainly because he wasn't under pressure to 'perform' or be something that he isn't; he was, and still is, encouraged to learn and develop the best that he can. As his mother, I couldn't ask for more. My son is happy and enjoys his school, and each day he surprises us with new words or skills. Billy is healthy, and now happy, thanks to the Whole Health Learning approach.

In the next chapter Jon will discuss some of the nutritional approaches that can help people with autism.

CHAPTER 10

Nutrition for Whole Health

Many people with autism have a very self-limiting diet which would not provide the diverse range of nutrients required by the body. Furthermore, many foods are deficient in nutrients as a consequence of over-farmed, nutrient-poor soil, and individuals with autism may have problems chewing, digesting and absorbing nutrients. I have worked with patients who eat such limited diets I honestly do not know how they have survived. One child would only eat custard cream biscuits, another drank 4.5 litres (8 pints) of milk each day, and another just ate marmite and bread. There are many such extreme cases, and countless others who live off refined carbohydrates, saturated fats, sugary foods, fizzy drinks, white bread, crisps, chips, cakes and biscuits with absolutely no intake of vegetables and fruit.

The Greek physician Hippocrates (460–377 BC) said, 'The natural healing force within each one of us is the greatest force in getting well. Our food should be our medicine. Our medicine should be our food.' In this chapter I shall be passing on ideas to help you support your child by providing the correct dietary advice about food sources and selection, nutrient-deficiency symptoms and how to improve them, as well as some simple tips on supplementation.

The human body is the greatest machine on earth. Like a high-performance car, it needs the correct type of fuel in the correct amounts to make it go. To run smoothly and last longer it needs high-quality fuel that's free from impurities.

The fuel to make our body work efficiently comes from the foods we eat, and how smoothly it runs depends on what's in that food and on how well we digest and absorb the nutrients and other beneficial components within it.

The marvellous thing about refuelling the human body is that food doesn't just provide the raw material for energy to keep our heart beating and our muscles working – although it does this incredibly efficiently. It also provides the body with all the microscopic building blocks it needs to carry out a staggering number of highly complex biochemical tasks every moment we're alive.

In this chapter I'll look at some of the specialist diets that may help to alleviate, or even eradicate, some of the symptoms of autism. The range of diets that are available, and those that have been used by parents for their children, continues to grow. This becomes increasingly problematical for parents when trying to decide which one is the most suitable for their child. This chapter will help you, with the guidance of a qualified nutritionist, to make the correct decision about which foods your child should consume to make up a diet that is specific to your child's individual requirements.

Eating for good health

As we've seen in previous chapters, the food we eat, and its component parts, are vital to all the body's functions. Foods provide the following essential nutrients:

- Proteins, which will be digested to form amino acids.
- Fats, lipids and the essential fatty acids, omegas-3, 6, 7 and 9.
- Carbohydrates, which will be digested to form sugars, especially glucose (which is brain fuel and for making cellular energy).
- Minerals; for example, calcium, magnesium and iron.

- Vitamins; for example, the fat-soluble vitamins A, D, E and K, and the water-soluble vitamins C and the B vitamins.
- Trace elements, such as selenium, manganese, molybdenum and chromium.
- Plant chemicals, such as bioflavonoids, and antioxidants such as quercetin.
- Fibre: both soluble and insoluble to support gut health and toxic elimination.
- Water for hydration (the body is approximately 72 per cent water).

All of these are vital ingredients for our own recipe for optimal health. We need them for many vital functions and requirements, including:

- To survive
- For growth
- To self-heal and repair the body
- To form structures such as muscle mass, bone tissue and organ tissue
- To provide energy for the body to utilise
- To assist in chemical reactions
- To make antioxidants, enzymes, hormones and neurotransmitters

When nutrients fall but the cocktail of contaminants rise

Unfortunately, much of our food also comes complete with a range of contaminants and noxious substances. Some of these occur quite naturally, but many more enter the food chain by being sprayed on crops, fed to livestock or added during processing, preparation or packaging. Over-farmed soils also lead to many foods being deficient in levels of certain nutrients.

This widespread and highly contentious issue is caused by modern intensive-farming methods, global food markets and (generally Western) shopping, cooking and eating habits. We have ourselves to blame to a large extent for a supermarket-dominated consumer culture that demands a vast range of sorted, processed and packaged foods shipped or flown in from all over the world, available all year round, consistent in colour, taste and texture and lasting for weeks. Consequently, our food may contain:

- Pesticides, herbicides, insecticides, antifungal agents
- Parasites, pathogenic bacteria, moulds
- E numbers, artificial colourings, flavourings, preservatives
- Components that feed gut bugs such as certain sugars (granulated, cane and maple syrup) and phenols (explained on page 230)
- Growth hormones and antibiotics, as found in non-organic meat and fish sources
- Fluoride, chlorine, heavy metals such as mercury, lead, aluminium

Natural toxins that are also found in food

A surprising number of generally harmless foods contain substances which, under certain conditions, or where present in certain parts of the plant, can be extremely harmful and should therefore be avoided in the diet. These include:

- Apple and pear pips (and the kernels of apricots, almonds, peaches, plums and cherries), which contain a substance called amygdalin. This interacts with enzymes and bacteria to form hydrogen cyanide in the gut. So don't chew the pips, or blend whole fruit.
- Cassava and bamboo shoots, which contain a similar substance to apple pips.

- Many plant foods (fruit and veg) contain organic acids called oxalates (oxalic acid) which bind to calcium, causing sharp crystals to form. This can cause abdominal pain and inflammation, pain on urination, oxidative damage (that is, damage to cells and structures caused by unstable molecules), glutathione depletion, vomiting and kidney stones. In high concentrations – for example in rhubarb leaves – oxalate poisoning can result in seizures and coma. In people with leaky gut, this toxicity can spread through the body.

- Salicylates are present in artificial food colourings and flavourings and in various concentrations in a great many plant foods that are otherwise healthy (such as fruits, veg, nuts, herbs and spices). Some people are sensitive to these compounds, or to some of the foods that contain them, which can lead to allergies or allergy-like symptoms, or to cognitive and perceptual disorders.

- Sweet potato, if damaged, produces a toxin called ipomeamarone, which gives the sweet potato a bitter taste and has been known to kill cattle (after eating a lot of it). It is recommended that you cut out any damaged parts of a sweet potato before cooking.

- Potatoes contain toxins called glycoalkaloids, similar to the poison in deadly nightshade (*Atropa belladonna*) from the same family of plants. The toxin is more concentrated in the leaves and stalks of the potato plant, and in sprouts from the tuber (the potato), and accumulate under the skin with age, exposure to light and damage; it is often associated with greening of the flesh of the potato. Poisoning can result in stomach cramps, headaches, diarrhoea and, in extreme cases, coma and death. Never eat the leaves or sprouts, and either completely cut out any green parts or discard greening potatoes.

- Lectins from red kidney beans can cause stomach cramps, vomiting and diarrhoea. Fresh or dry kidney beans should never be eaten raw, and should be soaked overnight then fast boiled in water for at least 10 minutes before simmering until cooked. Canned kidney beans are already treated to remove lectins.

There's no need to be alarmed by any of this. Most of the time, we get by without poisoning ourselves or causing great harm – and, for example, not eating green potatoes is just common sense. However, because many individuals with autism have problems removing toxins from the body, it is necessary to avoid putting more into the body. Many of the physiological and neurological symptoms we see in people with ASCs are remarkably similar to many of the effects of these toxins, and could be caused, prolonged or exacerbated by them.

Where do I start?

In my opinion, it is important that the specifics of a diet for someone with autism is taken very seriously, looked at extremely carefully and managed proactively through dietary intervention, nutritional and nutraceutical supplementation in order to improve their life.

Through my research and clinical experience I have come to the conclusion that many diets work on five simple main principles:

1. Choose organic

Use only organic, seasonal produce and foods free from additives, preservatives, flavourings, colouring, pesticides and fungicides.

This makes absolute sense for many reasons, not least the quite horrific litany of noxious or genetically modified substances that make their way into intensively farmed or processed foods. If sensitivities or detoxification problems exist, and one is trying to improve a child's abilities to eradicate toxins, it is obviously best to reduce toxic exposure via the food the child consumes (and to address the chemical content of *all* products used in the household).

An organic diet may have some drawbacks, such as increased levels of bacteria and fungi on the unprocessed fruits and vegetables consumed. Wash all fruit and veg well; peel fruits whenever possible.

Some foods are very high in pesticides and should therefore not be consumed unless they are organic: celery, peaches, strawberries, apples, blueberries, nectarines, peppers, spinach, kale and spring greens, cherries, potatoes, grapes, lettuce.

Not all non-organic fruits and vegetables have a high pesticide level. Some produce has a strong outer layer that provides a defence against pesticide contamination. The following foods contain little to no pesticides: onions, avocados, sweetcorn, pineapples, mango, peas, asparagus, kiwi fruit, cabbage, aubergine, cantaloupe melon, watermelon, grapefruit, sweet potatoes.

2. Avoid additives and go for preservative-free foods

Many individuals are extremely sensitive to chemicals added to foods, such as flavourings, colourings, preservatives, antifungals, antibacterials, E numbers, and so on. These also add a very toxic load to the body. Always read the label on packaged food. You will find plenty of information in books and on the Internet about additives and preservatives in food, but some of the main categories to avoid are as follows:

- Preservatives – particularly sodium benzoate
- Emulsifiers, stabilisers, thickeners and gelling agents
- Carrageenan
- Colourings – particularly tartrazine, E102, E165 and cochineal
- Anti-caking agents – particularly magnesium carbonate

- Flavourings and flavour enhancers
- Propylene glycol E1520 and MSG (monosodium glutamate)
- Artificial sweeteners – particularly aspartame

How vigilant you have to be when deciding which foods you must definitely avoid will greatly depend on which chemicals you discover your child has sensitivities to, but there is nevertheless something to be said for pursuing as natural a diet as possible. So, use the freshest organic produce, cook at home, wash vegetables and peel fruit as well as balancing your diet to include those foods that are required specifically by your child (I'll explain about these later).

3. Follow a hypo-allergenic diet

Remove all allergenic and opioid proteins from the diet, as these affect brain function. These foods include gluten and casein, and other compounds such as phenols, oxalates and salicylates that your child may be sensitive to. You will need to discover which foods are hypo-allergenic for your child by completing the home pulse test to identify the problem foods and then perhaps taking a blood sample and conducting a food antigen cellular test. The allergenic foods discovered by the tests are then taken out of the diet completely. Because an allergy is caused when the protein from these foods gets through the gut wall and enters the blood system, individuals with many food allergies must be checked for leaky gut as well as how efficient they are at digesting foods. An essential part of digestion is the correct amount of acids in the stomach; these trigger enzymes to be released which then digest the food. You can carry out the test below to see if your child has sufficient hydrochloric acid in the stomach:

Hydrochloric acid analysis:

Juice 115g (4oz) cooked beetroot (without added vinegar) and drink it on an empty stomach. Observe the urine for the following three hours and see if it shows any colouring from the beetroot. If colouring is found, it is likely that there are insufficient gastric secretions of hydrochloric acid and nutritional support may be necessary, such as vitamin B_6, zinc, digestive enzymes or betaine hydrochloride with pepsin or a combination of all of the above. Of course, the nutritional protocol for this must be decided upon by a qualified professional.

Testing for food allergies is also essential in selecting the correct food sources for your child. Look for outward symptoms of food allergy, such as red ear lobes, facial flushing, cravings for certain foods and hyperactivity shortly after consumption. If these are present, a simple pulse test for each individual food is described on page 60. Remember, food cravings may well be driven by those foods your child is allergic to, and sensitivities may also be caused by a zinc deficiency.

4. The diet must suit the gut ecology

There are a number of therapeutic diets – such as the specific carbohydrate diet, the anti-*Candida* diet and the body ecology diet – which starve pathogenic species of bacteria, fungi and moulds, thereby reducing their presence in the gut and reducing the toxins that are released by them. Phenolic compounds are an example of such organisms. They are used by particular bacteria in the gut to produce a potent neurotoxin called proprionic acid. A diet that avoids foods high in phenols will starve these bacteria and therefore reduce their numbers in the gut, and in turn reduce the harmful proprionic acid.

5. Eat foods that are nutrient dense

It is essential to identify the symptoms of nutrient deficiency – many individuals with an ASC are lacking sufficient levels of certain nutrients. A hair mineral analysis is one way to do this, or your practitioner can use the Nutreval or ONE test from

Genova Diagnostics, and I have also added a list which shows the symptoms of deficiencies in vitamins and minerals in the Appendix. Increase the range of foods that are richer in those nutrients that your child is lacking, as shown in the Appendix. Once the range of foods has been worked out, based on the above main principles, this will provide the basis for a diet that is appropriate for your child.

Drink plenty of water

Remember that it is essential to drink plenty of water, preferably purified – at least 1 litre (1¾ pints) per day.

Choosing the correct diet

There is a variety of specific diets and dietary advice available to address many of the features of autism, and I have mentioned some of them above. But, of course, no two individuals will have the same symptoms or requirements, so the appropriate nutritional protocol must be designed by a qualified and experienced professional around the specific needs of each individual; however, before the diet can be started, the gut must be functioning well with good digestion and absorption, if not it is pointless providing the correct foods if they cannot be digested and their nutrients released for absorption. Once the gut is functioning optimally, the appropriate diet can be selected.

This is not easy, however, because many of the diets available seem to overlap or even contradict each other in terms of which foods can and cannot be eaten. Foods that are seen to be incredibly good for one reason may turn out to be terribly bad for another. This is, of course, because each body is different, and each diet is designed to address specific issues from a certain hypothesis, based on what symptoms are present, as well as the existing diet, allergies and intolerances, and gastrointestinal and biomedical conditions. Some common diets that have been used for children with autism are explained below:

Gluten-free, casein-free diet (GFCF)

The GFCF diet is probably the best-known dietary intervention for those with an ASC. On the GFCF diet gluten (the protein in wheat, rye, barley, spelt, kamut and commercial oats) and casein (the protein in dairy) are completely removed. I think it is worth all individuals trying this diet with their child for at least three months to see if you notice improvements. A child that craves milk and dairy products, wheat-based products, such as bread, cakes, pasta and biscuits, and who is a picky eater and who exhibits staring spells and has an absent expression would, in my opinion, benefit from a GFCF diet. Parents report that when these proteins are taken out of the diet the child has better attention, has better eye contact and heightened learning skills. The Autism Research Institute in America reported that this diet is helpful for 65 per cent of children with an ASC.

Gluten and casein are an issue for many children on the autism spectrum, because many have problems digesting these proteins because of a lack of the necessary digestive enzymes. The undigested proteins are then absorbed through a leaky gut and act as morphine-like proteins called opioid peptides, creating a number of significant effects, including inflammation, allergenic responses and cognitive dysfunction.

In the initial stages, this can be a difficult diet to manage, as so many of the foods we take for granted are based on wheat and dairy (bread, wheat flour, pasta, milk and cheese in their natural form as well as being included in other products), and alternatives to these may not be so familiar or so easy to find; however, many parents will tell you that the results are worth the effort, and alternatives, including specifically gluten-free and casein-free products and recipes are increasingly available.

Gluten

Avoid the following gluten foods: barley, biscuits, breakfast cereals, bulgar wheat, cakes, dumplings, macaroni, oats, pasta, rye, shop-bought soups, spelt, stuffing, wheat.

Replace with millet, quinoa, buckwheat, rice, corn.

Casein

Avoid butter, cheese, cocoa, condensed milk, cow's milk and milk products, creams, evaporated milk, ice cream, lactose, whey, yoghurt.

Replace with almond or hazelnut milk, coconut milk, rice milk, soya milk, casein-free products.

Anti-*Candida* diet

This diet focuses on removing foods that allow the gut to be colonised by the yeast *Candida albicans*, which is widespread in people with autism. Overgrowth can be due to the overuse of antibiotics, low sec IgA antibody production and a low Th1 response. It is important to have this assessed by a qualified nutritional practitioner, but signs such as abdominal bloating, white tongue, red anal area, thrush, night sweats and cravings for sweets and refined carbohydrates, apples, grapes, plums and cherries, may point to a *Candida* problem which would benefit from this diet and/or the body ecology diet.

Avoid the following foods:

- **Aged cheeses**: casein derived from aged cheese and the moulds themselves encourage *Candida* growth.
- **Additives and preservatives**: many of these chemicals can disrupt the beneficial bacteria in the gut and allow the *Candida* yeast to flourish, so it's advisable to steer clear of processed foods as much as possible.
- **Chocolate and sugar**. *Candida* loves sugar, so *Candida* sufferers will often have sweet cravings.

- **Fruit**: although it is generally very good for us, the sugar content of certain fruits can feed the yeast infection in a person suffering the effects of *Candida* overgrowth or candidiasis, so avoid apples, grapes, cherries, raisins and plums, as they contain arabinose sugars, which are much favoured by *Candida*.

- **Glutinous foods**: even if your child is not following a gluten-free diet, avoid foods containing gluten while addressing a *Candida* infection – that is, anything made with wheat, rye, oats or barley. Otherwise the immune system will spend all of its time and energy combating these proteins instead of attacking the *Candida*.

- **Spices, curries and hot foods**. Curries and spicy foods can destroy the beneficial bacteria in the gut and allow the *Candida* yeast to flourish.

- **Nuts**: although generally OK, some nuts – such as peanuts – can hide mould, or can promote or exacerbate a *Candida* infection.

- **Mushrooms**: *Candida* loves to feed on mould and fungi, so avoiding mushrooms will help to restrict the growth of the infection.

- **Condiments**: tend to be high in sugar so they can feed a *Candida* infection. Stay away from ketchup, mayonnaise, salad dressing, mustard, horseradish, Worcestershire sauce and soy sauce.

Hypo-allergenic diet

Any substance that causes an allergic response should naturally be avoided at all costs, as these cause inflammation and topical, or atopic, symptoms as a result of an immune response. The trick is to find out which of many foodstuffs are causing the allergic response in the first place, as discussed previously, and then to remove them from the diet for at least six months, after which a further pulse test will determine whether they can then be reintroduced.

Low oxalate diet

Oxalates are naturally occurring toxins in a wide variety of plant foods and virtually all seeds and nuts. When ingested by humans they are capable of reducing the absorption of zinc, calcium, magnesium and iron. They cause oxidative damage, deplete glutathione levels and cause inflammation and kidney dysfunction.

The low oxalate diet is potentially tricky, as so many foods contain oxalates. It therefore necessitates a regime of supplements to support the process as well as the elimination of those foods from the diet. A qualified nutritional therapist will assist you.

Typically, a low oxalate diet will require limiting or excluding quite a wide range of foods high in oxalates:

Avoid aubergine, baked beans, peanut butter, celery, chard, dandelion greens, green beans, kale, leeks, mustard greens, okra, parsley, peppers, sweet potatoes, spring greens, spinach, courgettes, tofu, watercress, blackberries, blueberries, canned fruit cocktail, gooseberries, lemon peel, lime peel, orange peel, raspberries, rhubarb, strawberries, tangerines, chocolate, cocoa, tomato soup, peanuts, pecan nuts, soya bean crackers, wheatgerm.

Low phenol/low salicylate/Feingold diet

Phenols feed many bad bacteria in the gut, and children with high levels of proprionic acid will benefit from a low phenol diet. Salicylates are types of phenol. Under normal circumstances, phenols don't cause a problem because they are broken down by one of the body's most important detoxification pathways (called the sulphation pathway); however, as we have discussed previously, many children with autism are found to have a deficient sulphation pathway, and are low in 'free' sulphate. This results in being unable to properly process phenols, which then accumulate faster than the body can deal with them, causing a range of symptoms including hyperactivity, dark circles under the eyes, red face and ears, headaches, difficulty falling asleep, night waking, night sweats, bed-wetting, erratic or self-injurious behaviour such as head-banging, smelly head and bed, acrid stools, irritability, inappropriate laughter, hives and other skin conditions.

A diet that avoids phenols and salicylates (such as the Feingold diet) for a limited period – and which then keeps exposure as low as possible thereafter – will allow the body's detoxification system to catch up. This dietary step is often taken in combination with a GFCF diet.

Phenol

Avoid almonds, apples, apricots, bananas, berries, chocolate, cocoa, milk/cheese, most herbs and spices, mushrooms, oranges, peanuts, peppers, pickles, red grapes, tomatoes.

Salicylate

Avoid almonds, apricots, cherries, cucumbers, honey, nectarines, pickles, pineapple, plums, radishes, raspberries, tomatoes. Also avoid additives, such as flavourings, preservatives, emulsifiers, MSG, nitrites, food perfumes, sorbates and sulphites.

Specific carbohydrate diet (SCD)

The SCD diet is often helpful for addressing dysbiosis and severe digestive conditions, and when gastrointestinal symptoms persist after a while on a GFCF diet.

SCD involves removing certain foods that are rich in complex starches and sugars (disaccharides and polysaccharides) from the diet. These substances are poorly digested by children whose intestines lack carbohydrate-digesting enzymes (amylases and ptyalin) because of pancreatic insufficiencies and/or who have inflamed digestive systems. When ingested, the starches and sugars that are not properly broken down feed yeast and bacteria, creating greater inflammation and digestive problems. By removing specific carbs from the diet, these bacteria (such as Clostridia) and yeasts are effectively starved to death.

Avoid starchy foods such as potatoes, rice, pasta, bread, sweet potato, noodles; sugary foods such as cakes, biscuits, syrup, sweets, chocolate, ice cream, fizzy drinks, sugary cereals; any processed foods containing sugar, such as ketchup, canned baked beans, and so on.

Eat meals based around meat, eggs, fish, with most green vegetables and salad vegetables (broccoli, cabbage, kale, spinach, Brussels sprouts, beansprouts, onions, leeks, lettuce, green beans).

Body ecology diet

The body ecology diet is a very specific regime designed by the nutritionist Donna Gates to combat yeast infection and fungal overgrowth and to support the growth and function of beneficial bacteria in the gut. The diet involves many of the principles of the other diets listed above, particularly the anti-*Candida* diet and SCD, but with the addition of a selection of cultured and fermented foods, pre- and probiotics and the principles of food combining.

Common digestive problems in ASCs

When your practitioner decides on the most appropriate diet the following factors will also be taken into consideration:

Poor chewing

Sometimes, poor chewing can be a simple key to problems with digestion. If your child doesn't chew food well (20 chews or so before swallowing) especially when eating meat, this means the food isn't mashed by the teeth to break up the fibres. The enzymes in the mouth that start the digestive process aren't given time to do their work and the acids and enzymes in the stomach and intestines are having to work extra hard to digest large pieces of food. Check how well your child is chewing, and if it's a problem, start by cutting food into smaller pieces, or even puréeing it.

Is the stomach producing enough hydrochloric acid?

As mentioned on page 229, gastric acid in the stomach is a vital part of the digestive process, creating the right pH for stomach enzymes to work and killing off harmful bacteria in the food. You can test for this, as explained earlier.

Is the pancreas releasing sufficient digestive enzymes?

This is very difficult to ascertain without laboratory testing, but if there is undigested food in the stool then this may be an issue.

Is nutrient absorption good?

Recurrent diarrhoea is a good indicator that something is wrong, and the rapid transit time that this implies will almost certainly lead to, or exacerbate, malabsorption and nutrient deficiencies. The signs and symptoms of malabsorption vary widely depending on which particular enzymes or body systems are deficient, but the following is a rough guide: 'failure to thrive', fatigue, rashes, easy bruising, muscle cramps and joint pain may all be attributable to malabsorption; inadequate fat absorption may result in pale, soft and smelly, or floating, stools; poor sugar absorption can cause abdominal bloating, diarrhoea and wind. The Bristol Stool Chart on pages 51–2 is a simple way to keep track of digestive and absorption issues, and any recurrent problems should be investigated either by your doctor, or through a nutrient deficiency test such as the ONE test or Nutreval Test through your practitioner.

Does the child have allergies to foods?

Earlier I listed some outward symptoms of food allergy and on page 60 I listed the pulse test. There is also another test for finding allergies, called the FACTest.

How is the child's pH balance?

Optimum pH (about 7.4 – slightly alkaline) is vital to the proper functioning of nutrient digestion and absorption, energy production, detoxification and cell repair. In very general terms, healthy people have alkaline body fluids but those of sick people are acidic. It's relatively simple to test the pH in saliva (which is a good indicator of pH in the gut) and the urine (which is a good indicator of pH in the bloodstream) using litmus paper strips.

Some foods promote acid production (for example, fizzy drinks, whole wheat, red meat), and some increase alkalinity (for example, mineral water, poached eggs, spinach, cabbage, soft cheese, millet).

The need for supplementation

It is very common for individuals with an ASC to need additional support via nutritional supplements, especially if they are eating a limited number of foods or have poor digestion and absorption. Each individual will have differing symptoms and the practitioner will need to decide on the type of supplement, its components and its specificity in addressing the particular deficiencies and imbalances. The practitioner must also consider which form of supplement is most appropriate for the person taking it, whether capsule, tablet, liquid or powder.

How to give your child supplements

Giving your child supplements isn't easy. Children with an ASC often have to take many supplements a day – anywhere from 6 to 30 – and this can be very difficult for parents. The following information is based on the excellent guidelines by Lori Knowles in her online article 'Getting Children to Take Supplements'.

Below are some suggestions that have been tried and tested to help overcome the problem of children running away, clenched teeth or spitting back out what is put into their mouths. Whether the supplements you are giving are in capsule, liquid or chewable form, following these steps should help with getting your child to comply.

1. **Take a no-nonsense approach**. Give supplements with the same level of intensity that you use to give them a life-saving medication. Your child needs these supplements to support their brain, immune system and overall nutritional status. Your child can sense when you mean business and you cannot allow them to think that taking their supplements is optional.

2. **Do not mix into food or drink and pretend that it's not there!** They may taste it and this may further reduce their dietary intake and this is very important to those children who are already picky eaters.

3. **Choose the best method for your child to administer supplements**. You need to consider the sensory/swallowing issues that your child has. Does your child do better with liquids or semi-solids? The two most common mediums in which to mix supplements are baby fruit purées or 1 or 2 tablespoons of strong-tasting liquids. I mixed Billy's supplements with maple syrup. Other

liquids suitable to mix supplements in include: pear, pineapple, orange, or water. It is recommended that you only use 1–2 tablespoons of liquid and only use the liquid of choice for giving supplements, not for regular drinks in order to avoid confusion.

4. **Remember that the choice of liquids or purées used should be based upon your child's issues,** so you need to take into consideration any allergies, phenol sensitivities and sensitivity to sugar.

5. **Use the concept of 'first – then'.** This is a critical concept to ensure compliance. If your child is in an ABA programme (see page 144), this would be a good place to learn this concept. Otherwise, parents can reinforce this concept by repeating it in everyday life experiences, such as, first we turn on the water, then we wash our hands. Even a very young child can learn this concept if it's repeated enough. Once this concept is understood, you need to consistently use it to enforce compliance. Next, choose a favourite activity (eating the next meal, watching video/TV, favourite toy, blanket, and so on), for the purpose of withholding it until or *after* the child takes the supplements successfully. It is important to be *firm and never waiver* on this, because it will ensure that success will come quickly.

6. **Use rewards.** This comes in handy when a child needs extra reinforcement. Always give lots of praise and hugs as well as one good-tasting reward that they can associate with taking yucky supplements.

7. **Be consistent and firm.** If you are firm and do not give in over the conditions you set down for your child, most children will start to comply within two to three days, because they know that they cannot win the battle. Wait them out for as long as you need to, and when they finally

give in and take the supplements, quickly give them praise, the preferred activity and the small reward that is given every time they successfully take their supplements. This positive reinforcement will encourage them to be more willing next time.

Recognising health issues in your child is imperative, and utilising foods and supplemental nutrients will help you to provide the necessary ingredients for their body to heal itself. As you will now appreciate, there is a range of factors to be considered when treating ASCs, but with knowledge and the correct practitioner to support you on your journey, the light that was once at the end of a very long tunnel will become closer and brighter each day.

In the Conclusion, Polly looks forward with optimism to the future for Billy and all children with autism.

Conclusion – The Future

I happened to be chatting with Billy's principal of his fabulous school one day in the summer of 2007. Billy was 11 years old. 'What's going to happen to Billy when he leaves here at 17?' I asked casually.

The principal looked me in the eye and said, 'This is the biggest tragedy of all. I'm afraid the future for children like Billy is bleak. I spent years getting young men and women with autism to learn skills suitable for employment. They leave this school suited and booted and full of confidence. They return within six months – there is very little, if anything, out there for them.'

This was a huge shock to me. I assumed that as Billy had been so well educated this far that the level of care and ongoing education he had been receiving would naturally continue for the rest of his life. I immediately sent out 350 letters to random readers of the *Autism File* asking them what they knew about the future for our children – what happens to them when they become adults. The feedback was, quite frankly, frightening. There was without doubt a real problem with adult provision for autism.

I knew I had to do something for Billy, but it was also obvious from the emails and letters I was receiving that there were a great many people like him out there.

I had to think about what was realistically right and best for Billy. He had come a long way: we could now communicate with him; he knew what he wanted and would ask for anything he couldn't get himself. He was talented on the computer, Play-station and other such equipment. He had made things at school that showed us he had many skills that, with support, could be developed further. Could Billy survive in today's world with-out support? No, he couldn't. That's an honest answer from his parents. I would love to write that he could, but honesty will help Billy, whereas hoping and hiding does neither.

Provision for adults with autism

There are some excellent organisations that provide training combined with support for adults with autism. The problem is that because the autism spectrum is so huge, different kinds of support are always needed. If we are to believe the figures that are pointing to steeply rising numbers of children with autism in the UK, we need to make planning for their adult lives a priority *now*, as those few excellent organisations are not going to be nearly enough for our children in the future.

I visited some of the organisations that already work with adults: the Irish Society for Autism's fabulous Dunfirth Farm in Ireland; ESPA (Education and Services for People with Autism) in Sunderland; and The Hesley Group. All are excellent models of best practice for varying degrees of autism.

I set up The Autism Trust as there was nowhere that catered for children like Billy and their future. The goal at the Trust is to pro-vide residential and professional support for children in the UK with autism once they leave supported education. The Trust has developed a network of consistently outstanding and innovative outreach centres for autism.

Three years of research has gone into finding out what adults with autism want and need, with a view to setting up centres of excellence. The centres have been designed by parents and people with autism with the aim of providing services and sup-port for all those who need it.

Many people have joined our fundraising efforts to get the first centre open. Each Autism Trust centre will be open to the public. There will be a Wellness Centre to cater for people of all ages who need help and advice with nutrition, relaxation and counselling as well as other beneficial therapies. The Trust will also run business centres where people who are able to can run their own companies with as much support as they need; for example, there will be some people, like Billy, who may be able to test computer games for a number of hours per week. The business centres will give people the chance to develop any skills they may have.

There will also be a conference and training centre, which will be used for training the public sector – the police, teachers, carers, paramedics and GPs – in an understanding of all aspects of autism, from developmental to biomedical and behavioural.

Each centre will have a café and shop managed by people with autism. Adults with all different levels of autism will be able to make products to sell in the shop. The Trust will also enable us to work with the great many other autism charities that are already doing valuable work.

Hope for the future

For those with a newly diagnosed child, the future is a daunting prospect. Your energies will be taken up with what you are dealing with now, and you may feel alone; however, today things are very different from when we first discovered that Billy had an ASC, and we are now doing something important towards the future for all of our children.

If health, education and support are put in place for people like Billy at the very beginning of a diagnosis and it continues right through to adulthood, what we will have is a person who can give something very special back into life. At the beginning, we were apprehensive about what the future might hold for Billy, but I'm not frightened anymore about who or what Billy is – in fact I am proud. Billy is a gift, not to just Jon and me but to society. He has already taught us so much, and will continue to do so. We just need to accept – to learn and love. It has been, and still is, an incredible journey with Billy and the great many others who we meet and speak to – but knowing you are not on your own is everything.

We are already making great strides to improve the lives of people with autism. This is ongoing and will continue for some years – and somehow I just know that everything will be all right for Billy and our children.

As I write these last few lines, I stop and remind myself where we are. It's a rare warm, sunny day. The children are on half-term. Bella is 15; music blares from her room as she and a friend get ready to go shopping. Outside, I hear the happy banter of four boys kicking a football around. Twelve-year-old Toby and his two friends are frantically trying to outdo the goalie; the goalie is good – the goalie is Billy. Billy is 14, playing football and arguing whether it was a good shot or not. There is a smash, a crash, something is broken. Silence, followed by small laughter. Billy comes in:

'Sorry Mum, I broke a plant pot.' He looks worried.

'That's OK Billy, thank you for telling me,' I say.

Billy then goes and clears up the pieces and puts them in the bin. Within a few minutes he is back in goal.

I stop and think. We really have achieved so much with our boy. I didn't think I would ever hear his voice. Remember the day I would have given my right arm for him to touch his nose when asked? The day he didn't know his name or that I was his mother? The day he would have hit Bella if any noise was too loud? Those days are so far away. Billy has autism, but sometimes you just wouldn't even know.

Resources

Recommended reading

Blaxill, M. and Olmsted, D., *The Age of Autism: Mercury, Medicine, and a Man-made Epidemic*, Thomas Dunne Books, 2010

Bluestone, J., *The Fabric of Autism: Weaving the Threads into a Cogent Theory*, The Handle Institute, 2004

Bock, K., MD, Bock, S.J., MD and Faass, N., MSW, MPH, *The Germ Survival Guide*, McGraw-Hill, 2003

Bock. K., MD, Fink, K, and Stauth, C., *Healing The New Childhood Epidemics: Autism, ADHD, Asthma, and Allergies*, Ballantine Books, 2007

Bock, K., MD and Sabin, N., *The Road to Immunity: How to Survive and Thrive in a Toxic World*, Simon & Schuster, 1997

Bock, S.J., MD, Bock, K., MD and Bruning, N.P., *Natural Relief For Your Child's Asthma: A Guide to Controlling Symptoms & Reducing Your Child's Dependence on Drugs*, HarperCollins, 1999

Buckley, J.A., *Healing Our Autistic Children: A Medical Plan*, Palgrave Macmillan, 2010

Chauhan, A., Chauhan, V. and Brown, T. (eds), *Autism: Oxidative Stress, Inflammation, and Immune Abnormalities*, CRC Press, 2009

Clements, J., *People with Autism Behaving Badly: Helping People with ASD Move on from Behavioural and Emotional Challenges*, Jessica Kingsley, 2005

Clements, J. and Zarkowska, E., *Behavioural Concerns and Autistic Spectrum Disorders: Explanations and Strategies for Change*, Jessica Kingsley, 2000

Clements, J., Hardy, J. and Lord, S., *Transition Or Transformation? Helping Young People With Autistic Spectrum Disorder Set Out on a Hopeful Road Towards Their Adult Lives*, Jessica Kingsley, 2010

Converse, J., *Special-Needs Kids Eat Right: Strategies to Help Kids on the Autism Spectrum Focus, Learn, and Thrive*, Penguin, 2009

Davis, D., *Sound Bodies through Sound Therapy*, Kalco Publishing LLC, 2004

De Felice, K., *Enzymes: Go with your Gut*, Thundersnow Interactive, 2006

Delaine, S.K., *The Autism Cookbook*, Skyhorse Publishing, 2010

Gates, D., *Body Ecology Diet*, B.E.D. Publications, 2007

Gottschall, E.G., *Breaking the Vicious Cycle: Intestinal Health Through Diet*, Kirkton Press, 1994

Harper-Hill, K., and Lord, S., *Planning to Learn: Creating and Using a Personal Planner with Young People on the Autism Spectrum*, Jessica Kingsley, 2007

Herskowitz, V., *Autism & Computers: Maximizing Independence Through Technology*, AuthorHouse, 2009

Ingram, Dr C., *Nutrition Tests for Better Health*, Knowledge House, 2004

Jepson, B., *Changing the Course of Autism: A Scientific Approach for Parents and Physicians*, Sentient Publications, 2007

Kessick, R., *Autism and Diet: What You Need to Know*, Jessica Kingsley, 2009

Kessick, R., *Autism and Gastrointestinal Complaints: What You Need to Know*, Jessica Kingsley, 2009

Kirby, D., *Evidence of Harm*, St Martins Press, 2005

Lansky, A.L., *Impossible Cure: The Promise of Homeopathy*, R.L. Ranch Press, 2003

Le Breton, M., *Diet Intervention and Autism*, Jessica Kingsley, 2001

Lewis, L., *Special Diets For Special Kids I & II*, Future Horizons, 2001

Lord, R.S. and Brailey, J.A., *Laboratory Evaluations for Integrative and Functional Medicine*, Metametrix Institute, 2008

Lynch, B.M. and Rasmussen, T., *The Verbal Behavior Approach: How to Teach Children with Autism and Related Disorders*, Jessica Kingsley, 2007

Lyons, T., *1,001 Tips for the Parents of Autistic Girls*, Skyhorse Publishing, 2010

Marohn, S., *The Natural Medicine Guide to Autism*, Hampton Roads, 2002

Marsden, K., *Good Gut Healing*, Piatkus, 2003

Matthews, J., *Cooking To Heal: Autism Nutrition Cookbook and Instructional DVD*, Healthful Living Media, 2009

Matthews, J., *Nourishing Hope for Autism: Nutrition and Diet Guide for Healing Our Children*, Healthful Living Media, 2008

Maurice, C., *Let Me Hear Your Voice: A Family's Triumph over Autism*, Ballantine Books, 1994

McCandless, J., *Children with Starving Brains: A Medical Treatment Guide for Autism Spectrum Disorder*, 4th edn, Bramble Books, 2009

O'Brien, Robyn and Krantz, Rachel, *The Unhealthy Truth: How Our Food is Making Us Sick – and What We Can Do About it*, Broadway Books, 2009

Pitchford, P., *Healing with Whole Foods*, North Atlantic Books, 2002

Rimland, B., *Infantile Autism: The Syndrome and Its Implication for a Neural Theory of Behavior*, Prentice Hall, 1964

Rimland, B., Pangborn, J. and Baker, S., *2007 Supplement – Autism: Effective Biomedical Treatments (Have We Done Everything We Can for this Child? Individuality in an Epidemic)*, Autism Research Institute, 2007

Rimland, B., Pangborn, J. and Baker, S., *Autism: Effective Biomedical Treatments (Have We Done Everything We Can For This Child? Individuality In An Epidemic)*, Autism Research Institute, 2005

Robbins, J., *A Symphony in the Brain: The Evolution of the New Brain Wave Biofeedback*, Grove Press, 2008

Seroussi, K., *Unraveling the Mystery of Autism and Pervasive Developmental Disorders*, Simon & Schuster, 2000

Seroussi, K. and Lewis, L., *The Encyclopedia of Dietary Interventions for the Treatment of Autism and Related Disorders*, Sarpsborg Press, 2008

Silva, L., *Helping your Child with Autism: A Home Program from Chinese Medicine*, Guan Yin Press, 2010

Siri, K., *1,001 Tips for the Parents of Autistic Boys*, Skyhorse Publishing, 2010

Siri, K. and Lyons T., *Cutting-Edge Therapies for Autism*, Skyhorse Publishing, 2010

Stagliano, K., *All I Can Handle: I'm No Mother Teresa*, Skyhorse Publishing, 2010

Wakefield, A.J., *Callous Disregard: Autism and Vaccines – The Truth Behind a Tragedy*, Skyhorse Publishing, 2010

Wolfberg, P.J., *Play and Imagination in Children with Autism*, 2nd edn, Autism Asperger Publishing Company, 2009

Yasko, A., *Autism: Pathways to Recovery*, Neurological Research Institute, 2009

Yasko, A., *Genetic Bypass: Using Nutrition to Bypass Genetic Mutations*, Neurological Research Institute, 2005

Contact information

The Autism Trust UK and US charity committed to building
futures for people with autism. 45 Nightingale Road, Hampton,
Middlesex TW12 3HX; tel.: +44(0) 20 8783 3714;
www.theautismtrust.org.uk

Autism File A quarterly international magazine dealing with
all aspects of autism. 45 Nightingale Road, Hampton,
Middlesex TW12 3HX; tel.: +44(0) 20 8979 2525; www.autismfile.com

The Autism Clinic A nutritional clinic that specialises in the
treatments of health conditions and autism. 45 Nightingale Road,
Hampton, Middlesex TW12 3HX; tel.: +44(0) 7714 957309;
www.theautismclinic.com

ACT Today! (Autism Care & Treatment Today!) is a non-profit
organisation whose mission is to provide funding and support to
families that cannot afford the treatments their children with
autism need to achieve their full potential. 19019 Ventura Blvd. Suite
200, Tarzana, CA 91356; tel.: (818) 705 1625; Info@act-today.org

AutismOne A non-profit, charity organisation educating more than
100,000 families every year about prevention, safety and change.
1816 W. Houston Avenue, Fullerton, CA 92833; tel.: (714) 680 0792;
www.autismone.org

Autism Research Institute is devoted to conducting research and
to disseminating the results of research on the triggers of autism
and on methods of diagnosing and treating it. 4182 Adams Avenue,
San Diego, CA 92116; tel.: (619) 281 7165; Contact: Matt Kabler:
matt@autism.com; www.autism.com/

National Autism Association (NAA) raises funds for autism
research and support, and also provides programmes, such as
Helping Hand, Family First, and FOUND, designed to aid specific
needs for families dealing with autism. 1330 W. Schatz Lane, Nixa,
MO 65714; tel.: (877) 622 2884; naa@nationalautism.org;
www.nationalautism.org

SafeMinds is an organisation dedicated to research and awareness of mercury's involvement in such neurological disorders as autism, attention deficit disorder, and more. 16033 Bolsa Chica St. #104-142, Huntington Beach, CA 92649; tel.: (404) 934 0777; www.safeminds.org/

Talk About Curing Autism (TACA) provides medical, diet and educational information geared towards children with autism, and the organisation also has support, resources and community events. 3070 Bristol Street, Suite 340, Costa Mesa CA 92626; tel.: (949) 640 4401; (949) 640 4424; www.tacanow.org

The Autism Hope Alliance ignites hope for families facing the diagnosis through education and funding to promote progress now. 752 Tamiami Trail, Port Charlotte, FL 33953; tel.: (888) 918 1118; info@autismhopealliance.org

Unlocking Autism was created to find information about autism and disseminate that information to families of children with autism. The organisation also raises funds for research and awareness. P. O. Box 208, Tyrone, GA 30290; tel.: (866) 366 3361; www.unlockingautism.org

Child Early Intervention Medical Center, FZ LLC Al Razi Building, Block B, Suite 2010, Dubai Health Care City, P.O. Box 505122, Dubai, UAE; tel: +971 4 423 3667; fax: +971 4 429 8474; mobile: +971505512319; www.childeimc.com

MINDD Foundation was created to inform and provide research findings on new and alternative treatments for disorders like autism, such as chiropractic care, Chinese medicine and holistic care. PO Box 151 Vaucluse, NSW 2030, Australia; tel.: +61 2 9337 3600; info@mindd.org; www.mindd.org

Autism South Africa is the recognised, authoritative and representative national body that endeavours to ensure a meaningful quality of life for all people with an ASC in South Africa. P. O. Box 84209, Greenside, 2034, South Africa; tel: +27 11 484 9909;

fax: +27 11 484 3171; info@autismsouthafrica.org;
www.autismsouthafrica.org

Education

Autism Center for Enlightenment was founded in September of
2005 to make parents, government decision makers and medical
professionals aware of the growing evidence that autism is a
treatable, medical illness. Naperville, Illinois 60563;
info@autismcenterforenlightenment.com;
www.autismcenterforenlightenment.com

Autism Human Rights & Discrimination Initiative is a task
force that was created to address human rights violations and
discrimination against persons with autism and other cognitive
challenges internationally. Visit www.autismdiscrimination.com

Kenneth Bock MD Rhinebeck Health Center and The Center for
Progressive Medicine, Rhinebeck, 108 Montgomery Street,
Rhinebeck, NY 12572; www.rhinebeckhealth.com

Boston Higashi School 800 North Main Street, Randolph,
MA 02368; tel.: (781) 961 0800; www.bostonhigashi.org

CARD (Center for Autism and Related Disorders, Inc) 19019
Ventura Blvd, Suite 300, Tarzana CA, 91356; tel.: (818) 345 2345;
info@centerforautism.com; www.centerforautism.com

LVS Hassocks A new school, located near Brighton, specifically
for children with learning difficulties, such as autism, Asperger's
syndrome and dyslexia. London Road, Sayers Common, West
Sussex BN6 9HT; tel.: +44(0) 1273 832901; www.lvs-hassocks.org.uk

Parents for the early intervention of Autism (Peach) are the
fastest growing UK parent-led charity established to promote Early
Intensive Behavioural Intervention (EIBI) for young children with
autism, often referred to as applied behavioural analysis (ABA).
Whether you are a parent of a child with autism, a professional,

a practitioner already in this field, or quite simply interested, this website will:

- Introduce you to autism and give you guidance on obtaining a diagnosis.
- Talk about early behavioural intervention and how it could work for your child.
- Introduce you to the work of Peach and invite you to become a Peach member.
- Explain how they support tutors and established practitioners as well as parents.
- Inform you about training and resources that will develop your skills and knowledge.
- Give you hope for the future of your child.

The Brackens, London Road, Ascot, Berkshire, SL5 8BE; www.peach.org.uk

Pyramid Educational Consultants UK Ltd The official provider of the Picture Exchange Communication System (PECS) and the Pyramid Approach to training in the UK and Ireland.
Tel: +44(0) 1273 609555; www.pecs.org.uk

Son-Rise Program A treatment for autism, pervasive development disorder, Asperger's syndrome and other developmental disorders.
Tel.: +1(877) 766 7473 or +1(413) 229 2100;
www.autismtreatmentcenter.org

Supplements and testing services

Ainsworths Pharmacy 36 New Cavendish Street, London W1G 8UF;
tel.: +44(0) 207 935 5330; www.ainsworths.com

BeginningwithA is an independent consultancy offering quality training and diagnostic services for professionals and for people affected by autism. Tel.: +44(0) 1223 633695;
enquiries@beginningwitha.com; www.beginningwitha.com

Candice Joyce RS Hom, Homeopathic Practitioner, Green Daises, 2 Gould Road, Twickenham TW2 6RS; tel.: 0781 8070754; Candice@greendaises.co.uk

Genova Diagnostics, Individual WellBeing Diagnostic Laboratories, Parkgate House, 356 West Barnes Lane, New Malden, Surrey KT3 6NB; tel.: +44 (0) 20 8336 7750; infouk@gdx.net

Laboratoire Philippe Auguste Specialising in preventive medicine. 119 Avenue Philippe Auguste, 75011 Paris; tel.: +33 1 43 67 57 00; fax: +33 1 43 79 00 27; contact@labbio.net; www.labbio.net

Great Plains Laboratory Provides urine testing and analysis for autism and other conditions. Tel.: +1(913) 341 8949; www.greatplainslaboratory.com

Metametrix Laboratory Tel. (Int): +1 8002214640; tel. (UK): +44(0) 80 8234 1629; www.metametrix.com

Products without chemicals and for specific diets

Dietary Needs Direct supplies an extensive range of products that are free from gluten, wheat, dairy and other allergens, for people with intolerances, allergies or on special diets. They specialise in GFCF food (autism spectrum) as well as covering anti-*Candida*, SCD(TM), coeliac and vegan diets among others. Each product is clearly flagged for its suitability and it is possible to shop by diet, by section, by product group or to quick shop from the website. Orders are also taken by phone, fax or email. Fairfield Court Units, Fairfield, Bromsgrove, B61 9NJ; tel.: +44(0) 1527 570444; www.dietaryneedsdirect.co.uk

GoodnessDirect Dietary options for products suitable for your diet. Tel.: +44(0) 87 1871 6611; www.goodnessdirect.co.uk

Green People Organic products made using mild natural ingredients so they are suitable for everyone, with dedicated ranges for men, women, babies and children. They don't use: lanolin, petrochemicals, propylene glycol, parabens, colourants

or fragrances. 10–11 Pondtail Farm, Coolham Road,
West Grinstead, RH13 8LN; tel.: +44(0) 1403 740350;
fax: +44(0) 1403 741810; Organic@greenpeople.co.uk

Online sources

Age of Autism is an online blog with daily news on the latest autism
research, updates and community happenings.
www.ageofautism.com/

Autism Canada Foundation www.autismcanada.org/

Directgov for information on education
www.direct.gov.uk/choosingaschool

EmergenzAutismo (Italy) www.emergenzautismo.org/

Schafer Autism Report is an online publication covering autism-
related issues.
edit@doitnow.com; www.sarnet.org/

Facebook groups
www.facebook.com/autismfile
www.facebook.com/autismfile.mothers
www.facebook.com/autismfile.wakefield
www.facebook.com/autismfile.sibs
www.facebook.com/autismtrust.campaign2010

Twitter
www.twitter.com/pollytommey
www.twitter.com/autismfile

Appendix

The charts on the following pages show good natural sources of vitamins and minerals and the physical signs of any deficiencies. The lists are for your information and are intended to prepare you for the possibly complex nutritional protocol that your practitioner will prescribe for your child.

VITAMINS

What does this vitamin do?	Good sources	Deficiency signs and symptoms
Vitamin A (retinol from meat sources and carotenoids from vegetable sources)		
Vitamin A is essential for the health and structure of the skin and mucous membranes (such as, in the nose, lungs and digestive tract). It is an antioxidant and is good for strengthening the immune system and for vision in low light conditions. Plant sources, such as beta-carotene must be converted to vitamin A in the body.	Cheese, eggs, liver, kidneys, oily fish, milk, yoghurt, orange fruit and veg, such as carrots, pumpkin, mango, apricots, and green veg, such as kale and spinach. It is also added to some low-fat spreads. Liver is such a rich source of vitamin A that the FSA recommends limiting the amount you eat, and advises that pregnant women should avoid it.	Red, itchy eyes, night blindness, sensitivity to bright lights, rough or dry skin, cold or infections, especially respiratory tract, allergies, acne.
Vitamin D (cholecalciferol and ergocalciferol)		
Vitamin D is processed into a hormone via the liver and kidneys and acts to regulate the amount of calcium absorbed by the	The majority of the vitamin D our body needs is obtained from the action of ultra-violet rays from sunlight on our skin.	Soft teeth/tooth decay, fatigue, short sightedness, loss of appetite, insomnia, visual problems, diarrhoea, burning

intestines (making it available to build healthy bones). It is also vital in the process of cell division.

It is not abundant in food sources but occurs naturally in some, such as oily fish, meat, eggs and butter, and is added to fortify some fat spreads and cereal products.

sensation in mouth and throat.

Vitamin D deficiency can lead to serious skeletal deformity in children (rickets – childhood osteomalacia) and to pain and bone weakness in adults (osteomalacia).

Vitamin E (a group of compounds called tocopherols, especially alpha tocopherol)

Vitamin E supports the immune system, helps to suppress inflammation and is an antioxidant, i.e. it acts to protect cells against oxidative damage by free radicals.

Almonds, nut oils, sunflower seeds (and oil), corn (maize), peanuts (and peanut butter), spinach and olive oil.

Poor wound healing, inflamed veins, haemolytic anaemia, menstrual problems (mother), miscarriage, infertility, sterility (mother).

Deficiency is rare, and problems only tend to occur in people who have underlying metabolic disorders that prevent or impair the absorption of fats.

Vitamins chart continues

What does this vitamin do?	Good sources	Deficiency signs and symptoms
Vitamin K (vitamin K_1 – phylloquinone from plants and K_2 – menaquinone from animal sources)		
Vitamin K_1 is necessary for the healing of wounds as it aids the clotting of blood. It is also an important anti-inflammatory and helps prevent bone loss. K_2 helps the absorption of calcium by bone and thereby helps to prevent osteoporosis.	Green leafy vegetables such as kale, broccoli, Brussels sprouts, asparagus, Swiss chard, turnip greens and spinach. It is also available (in smaller quantities) in peas, carrots, some meats (such as pork and liver) and dairy products (such as cheese).	Poor liver function, nose bleeds, coeliac/ irritable bowel syndrome. Deficiency is rare. Newborn babies are prone to vitamin K deficiency as it doesn't cross the placenta, and gut flora haven't yet built up.
Vitamin C (ascorbic acid)		
Vitamin C is essential to the synthesis of collagen, an important component of blood vessels, ligaments, tendons and bones. It is an effective antioxidant, helps maintain healthy teeth and gums, plays an important role in the absorption of iron to make red blood cells, the synthesis of the mood hormone norepinephrine, and helps the conversion of fat molecules into energy.	Found in most fruit and vegetables, but sweet peppers, carrots, broccoli, sweet potato, watercress, oranges, grapefruit, lemons, blackcurrants, guava, papaya, melon, mango, Brussels sprouts and kiwi fruit are particularly excellent sources.	Common colds and infections, allergies, bleeding or inflamed gums, defective teeth, anaemia, easy bruising, loss of appetite, fatigue, anxiety, depression, slow wound healing, poor digestion. Severe deficiency can lead to the potentially fatal disease scurvy.

Vitamin B₁ (thiamin)

Thiamin (along with the other B vitamins) is needed to release the energy from carbohydrates – the more carbohydrate consumed, the more thiamin is needed. It is also instrumental in the normal function of the heart and nervous system.

Sunflower seeds, tuna, sweetcorn, lentils, pork, most vegetables, cheese, milk, fruit, eggs, wholegrain bread, and fortified cereal products.

Irritability, sensitivity to noise, anxiety and confusion, hypothyroidism, fear, constipation, fatigue, gastrointestinal disturbances, muscle loss, pins-and-needles, loss of appetite.

Vitamin B₂ (riboflavin)

Riboflavin is needed to release the energy from fat, protein and carbohydrate. It enables the transport and metabolism of iron and aids the structure of the skin and mucous membranes (such as in the lungs, intestinal tract and nose).

Liver, mushrooms, venison, shellfish, soya, almonds, beans, spinach, beef, cow's milk, goat's milk and fortified cereals.

Mouth and lip lesions especially at corners, tongue inflammation, gritty eyes/red itchy eyes, scaly skin on face/dermatitis, hair loss, insomnia, slowed mental response.

Any deficiency is usually associated with deficiency of all B vitamins.

Vitamins chart continues

What does this vitamin do?	Good sources	Deficiency signs and symptoms
Niacin (vitamin B₃)		
As with the other B vitamins, niacin is required to release the energy from protein, carbohydrates and fat. It also serves to lower overall cholesterol and triglycerides in the blood.	Niacin is found in many foods and can be synthesised in the body from the amino acid tryptophan. Yeast (such as marmite), beef, poultry, red fish (such as tuna and salmon), shrimp, spinach, liver, green leafy veg, prunes, dates and fortified cereals, are all good food sources. Also found in peanuts, legumes, lentils and coffee.	Eczema, diarrhoea, bad breath, fatigue, indigestion, depression, insomnia, skin eruptions, inflammation. Severe deficiency causes the disease pellagra, characterised by dermatitis, dementia and diarrhoea, and can be fatal.

Vitamin B6 (pyridoxine)

Vitamin B6 is vital to the use and storage of energy from carbohydrates and proteins. It is essential to the manufacture of red blood cells and for the function of the nervous system. It is involved in cell replication, digestion and antibody production and has a role in the regulation of mental processes and mood.

Vitamin B6 is found in a range of protein-rich meat and vegetable sources, especially chicken, fish, liver, kidney, pork, eggs, brown rice, milk, soya beans, wheatgerm, peanuts and walnuts.

Linear nail ridges, impaired wound healing, inability to tan, sensitivity to sun, cracks around lips, impaired memory, convulsions/tremors/seizures, hypoglycaemia, learning difficulties, diabetes, appetite loss, allergies, oedema (water retention), flaky skin, carpal tunnel syndrome (mother), irritability and depression, weakness, insomnia, hypersensitivity to noise.

Biotin (vitamin B7/vitamin H)

Biotin is a vital part of the process of 'extracting' the energy from fats and proteins – synthesising glucose from fatty acids and amino acids.

Egg yolks, cheese, liver, pork, salmon, avocados and mixed dried fruit.

Eczema and dermatitis, lack of appetite, lethargy, muscle aches and pains, cradle cap (dry scaly scalp), inflammation, pallor of skin, sore tongue.
Deficiency is extremely rare, as biotin is quite common and only needed in tiny amounts.

Vitamins chart continues

What does this vitamin do?	Good sources	Deficiency signs and symptoms
Folate (folic acid, vitamin B$_9$)		
Folate interacts with vitamin B$_{12}$ in the formation of red blood cells and is important in reducing the risk of certain birth defects such as spina bifida.	Folate is only found in small quantities, but in a wide range of foods. Liver, marmite, broccoli, Brussels sprouts, asparagus, spinach, peas, chickpeas, brown rice, and sunflower seeds.	Megaloblastic anaemia, depression, psychosis, epileptic fits, lack of appetite, sore red tongue, digestive disturbances, fatigue, insomnia, paranoia, memory problems.
Vitamin B$_{12}$ (cobalamin Cbl)		
Vitamin B$_{12}$ is important in making red blood cells and in the maintenance of the nervous system. It has a role in synthesising glucose energy from foods and is important to healthy growth and development in children. B$_{12}$ is also vital to the processing and use of folic acid (folate).	Virtually all meat and dairy products contain vitamin B$_{12}$. Most meats, salmon, cod, milk, cheese, eggs, yeast extract (such as marmite) and many fortified breakfast cereals and soya mince products. Seaweed (kelp) and sprouts are the only significant plant sources.	Abnormal gait/walking difficulties, pernicious anaemia, heart palpitations, loss of coordination (ataxia), impaired memory, sharp mood swings, constipation, digestive disorders, moodiness, hallucinations, ringing in ears. Deficiency is rare, but more common in elderly people and those on a vegan diet.

MINERALS

What does this mineral do?	Good sources	Deficiency signs and symptoms
Calcium		
Calcium is necessary for the growth and maintenance of strong bones, teeth and cell walls. It is an important component in blood clotting and helps to regulate muscle contraction – including the heartbeat. It is also thought that calcium helps to lower high blood pressure.	Around 70% of the calcium in the Western diet comes from milk, cheese and yoghurt. Cabbage, broccoli, walnuts, sesame and sunflower seeds, and soya beans are good vegetable sources. Whole fish (including bones – such as sardines). Bread and baked products are good because all flour (except wholemeal) in the UK is fortified with extra calcium. There is also calcium in drinking water.	Hyperactivity, fractures of bone, nervousness, muscle aches, leg cramps, teeth grinding, brittle nails, eczema, insomnia, pasty complexion, convulsions, cold sores, mouth blisters, impaired growth, high lead levels, high oxalic acid levels, poor fat digestion, abnormal heart rhythm.

Minerals chart continues

What does this mineral do?	Good sources	Deficiency signs and symptoms
Chloride/sodium chloride		
Chloride is a salt that the body uses for the production of stomach acids that are vital to digestion. It also helps to maintain a proper balance of body fluids.	The most common form of chloride is in table salt or sea salt – sodium chloride. It is found in vegetable sources such as tomatoes, celery, lettuce, olives, rye (grain) and seaweed. About 90% of salt intake comes from processed foods.	It is rare to be deficient in salt intake as it is so widely available in so many foods. Deficiency can occur with extreme fluid loss from prolonged vomiting or diarrhoea and can cause low blood pressure, dehydration, irritability and muscle cramps.
Iron		
Iron is essential for the production and maintenance of the haemoglobin in red blood cells, which is responsible for transporting oxygen around the body. It is also required for the functioning of many of the body's enzymes.	Good sources of iron include liver, meat, poultry and fish, nuts, beans and pulses, dried fruit, soya beans, kale, okra and watercress. Flour and many breakfast cereals are fortified with iron. Tea, coffee and spinach contain a substance that makes it difficult for the body to absorb iron.	Iron deficient anaemia, pallor, weakness and lethargy, shortness of breath, attention difficulties, brittle nails and hair, spoon-shaped nails or ridges running lengthwise, nervousness, slowed mental reactions.

Magnesium

Magnesium is vital for the function of the enzymes that break down nutrients to release energy; it is also important to cell metabolism and cell division; it is needed to enable vitamin D to do its work and for the parathyroid glands to produce and secrete hormones needed for bone health.

Magnesium exists in varying quantities in all foodstuffs. Rich sources include Brazil nuts, almonds, cashew nuts, roasted pumpkin seeds, bran cereal, spinach, quinoa and halibut. Other good sources include beans, tuna, peanuts, okra, pinenuts, pollock and soya beans.

Irregular/rapid heart beat, jumpy nerves, weak/twitching muscles, convulsions and seizures, fatigue, bed wetting, irritability, insomnia, depression, imbalanced pH, premature labour (mother), PMS (mother). Magnesium deficiency is linked to various disorders of the cardiovascular, gastrointestinal and central nervous systems, and to skeletal (bone) problems.

Phosphorus

Phosphorus works with calcium, in the form of calcium phosphate, in the development of healthy bones and teeth. It is required by every cell in the body and plays an important role in the metabolisation – energy release – of proteins, carbohydrates and fats.

Phosphorus is found widely in foods, usually combined with oxygen in the form of phosphates. Red meat is the richest source; other good sources include skimmed milk and dairy products, fish, poultry, bread and cereal products, eggs and rice.

Phosphorus is so widely available that deficiency is rare. Starvation, anorexia and alcoholism can result in phosphorus deficiency, with symptoms such as bone weakness and deformity, loss of appetite, vulnerability to infection and numbness in extremities.

Minerals chart continues

What does this mineral do?	Good sources	Deficiency signs and symptoms
Potassium		
Potassium works with sodium to maintain optimum pressure in the body's cells, which is vital for the transmission of nerve impulses and making muscles (such as the heart) work. Potassium is also instrumental in the function of some enzymes.	Potassium is present in all plant and animal tissues in various levels. Good sources include milk, most fruit (especially bananas) and veg, fish, shellfish, beef, liver, chicken and turkey. Potassium chloride is also used as an alternative to ordinary salt in low sodium table salt and processed foods.	Cognitive impairment, oedema (water retention), hypertension, irregular heart beat, nervousness and fatigue, abnormally dry skin, insomnia, nausea and vomiting, proteinuria (protein in urine). Potassium deficiency can result from loss of the mineral through severe vomiting, diarrhoea or other extreme fluid loss. In some cases, extremely low-calorie diets can lead to deficiency. Symptoms include irregular heartbeat, nausea, diarrhoea and weakness.

Sulphur

Sulphur exists in every cell. It has an essential role in the metabolism of proteins needed for growth and repair of body tissues such as cartilage and in the production of some enzymes. It is involved in the removal of some harmful substances from the body. There is limited evidence for a role for sulphur in skin health despite its use as a spa treatment.

Most of the sulphur that the body needs is metabolised from sulphur-containing amino acids in protein. It is also found, in the form of sulphites and sulphates, as food additives in some processed foods.

Dry hair, brittle nails, rough skin, pale stools, many bacterial infections, leaky gut, low glutathione levels.

Boron

Boron is known to be essential for humans, but its precise function is not known. It is thought that boron has a role in the metabolism and use of various other elements such as copper, calcium, magnesium, glucose, oestrogen and triglycerides (in fatty acids).

Boron is usually found in compounds such as borate, boric acid and borax and is present in many foods. Good sources are almonds, hazelnuts, cashew nuts, Brazil nuts and peanut butter; apricots, avocado, apples, tomatoes, kidney beans, dates and prunes.

Little is known about the effects of boron deficiency although it seems to affect calcium and magnesium metabolism. There is also some suggestion of a link with a musculoskeletal deficiency called Kashin-Beck Disease (KBD) which can lead to stunted growth and severe joint deformity.

Minerals chart continues

What does this mineral do?	Good sources	Deficiency signs and symptoms
Chromium		
Chromium enhances the effects of the hormone insulin and therefore affects the metabolism of glucose energy from carbohydrates, fats and proteins. It is also attributed with some beneficial effects on adult-onset diabetes and is associated in some studies with decreased body fat.	Dietary chromium is in a form called 'trivalent chromium' and is found in a variety of foods including (good sources) meats, whole-grain products, pulses (such as lentils), bran cereals, potatoes, brewer's yeast (supplements and beer) and spices.	Fatigue, anxiety, hypertension, impaired glucose metabolism, obesity. Deficiency is rare.
Cobalt		
Cobalt is an essential trace element that is a major constituent of vitamin B_{12}, so has a role in the metabolism of folate and fatty acids.	Cobalt is part of the structure of vitamin B_{12}, so adequate intake of foods rich in vitamin B_{12} will provide sufficient cobalt.	Cobalt deficiency has not been identified in humans, but any deficiency would be associated with vitamin B_{12} deficiency.

Copper

Copper plays an important part in the development of red blood cells by 'triggering' the release of iron from foodstuffs to form haemoglobin. It is vital for infant growth, the metabolism of glucose and cholesterol and has a role in brain and immune system development, connective tissue and bone structure.

Liver, oysters, crab, lobster, mushrooms (especially shiitake), dark chocolate, chestnuts, buckwheat, sunflower seeds, quinoa, asparagus, almonds and walnuts.

Deficiency is rare, and is most likely to arise from an underlying heath condition. Symptoms include anaemia, white blood cell depletion and bone abnormalities.

Fluoride

Fluoride is only considered an essential trace element due to its undeniable role in the prevention of dental caries (tooth decay). Fluoride is only found in the bones and teeth where it fills gaps between microscopic crystals of calcium and phosphate and so increases bone and tooth density.

Much of the fluoride intake of the general public comes from the synthetically produced fluoride used in toothpaste and mouthwash. Some areas of the UK (10–15%) have fluoride added to tap water. Good food sources include tea, marine fish with bones (such as sardines), other fish, chicken and grape juice.

Bacteria in dental plaque can metabolise certain carbohydrates (sugars), converting them to acids that can dissolve tooth enamel. Untreated tooth decay can lead to spreading infections, pain and tooth loss.

Minerals chart continues

What does this mineral do?	Good sources	Deficiency signs and symptoms
Iodine		
Iodine is a major component of the thyroid hormones thyroxin and triiodothyronine that help to regulate the body's metabolic rate, maintain cell health and are involved in the development of the nervous system.	Marine fish and shellfish are rich sources of iodine. It is present in kelp (seaweed) and in many cereals and grains, but levels vary according to the levels in the soil where they grow. Cow's milk also contains some iodine; possibly due to its use in cattle feed supplements and as a sterilising agent.	Goitre (thyroid swelling), obesity, dry hair, heart palpitations, a cold body, constipation, weakness, low resistance to colds and infections, nervousness, irritability. More severe deficiency can lead to hyperthyroidism. Severe deficiency in the developing foetus can cause cretinism – mental retardation, deaf-mutism and spastic diplegia.
Manganese		
Manganese is a component of some essential enzymes and is also involved in activating some enzymes responsible for the metabolism of carbohydrates, amino acids and cholesterol. Manganese is also involved in the production of collagen, which is vital for wound healing.	Pineapple is a particularly good source of manganese, as is tea. Other sources include pecan nuts, almonds and peanuts, kale, spinach, peas, runner beans, brown rice, bran and oatmeal cereal products, soya beans and potatoes.	Deficiency is rare and has only been observed experimentally (i.e. on purpose). Only minor symptoms were observed, such as slower fingernail growth and mild dermatitis.

Molybdenum

Molybdenum is a component and/or activator of some enzymes involved with the metabolism of sulphur-containing amino acids, uric acid and of genetic material (RNA and DNA) and aids the antioxidant capacity of the blood.

Nuts are good sources of molybdenum. It is present in plants that grow above ground, such as peas, leafy vegetables such as kale, spinach and cauliflower, cereals, etc. Plants grown in neutral or alkaline soils have higher concentrations.

Predisposition to tooth decay, anaemia, mouth and gum disorders. There is little evidence of deficiency in otherwise healthy people.

Selenium

Selenium is an important antioxidant – protecting the body from oxidative stress and damage from free radicals. It also plays an important role in the immune system, and in the production and metabolism of thyroid hormones.

Brazil nuts are a particularly good source of selenium, as is tuna and cod, beef, turkey, cottage cheese, bread and eggs. It is present in most meat, fish and nuts.

Susceptibility to colds/infections, fatigue, heart disease, pancreatic insufficiency. Selenium deficiency is linked to a heart muscle disorder called Keshan disease, causing an increase in heart size that can lead to heart failure.

Minerals chart continues

What does this mineral do?	Good sources	Deficiency signs and symptoms
Silicon		
Silicon is important to the maintenance of healthy bones and connective tissues in organ structure, tendons, ligaments and cartilage.	Silicon is found in highest concentrations in cereal grains, particularly oats, barley and rice. Beer is also a rich source. Water also contains silicon.	Silicon deficiency is not known in humans. In animal studies deficiency has been shown to affect joint and bone development.
Zinc		
Zinc is a vital component of many enzymes and is necessary for the metabolism of carbohydrates, fats and protein. It is also involved in cell production, wound healing and in the synthesis and regulation of genetic material.	Oysters, crab, lobster, beef, pork, chicken, baked beans, milk, cheese, yoghurt, cashew nuts, almonds, chickpeas, bread and wheat germ.	Slow learning, susceptibility to infections, loss of appetite, fatigue, loss of taste and smell, allergies, acne and dermatitis, white spots on nails, peeling, thin nails, impaired night vision, memory impairment, skin lesions, slow wound healing.

Below are some common symptoms associated with autism with the possible cause and the nutrients that may be required to support them, to give you an idea of what may be involved. You should not attempt to self-diagnose, however, but should seek advice and direction from a qualified nutritional practitioner if your child presents any of the symptoms.

Symptoms and their possible causes and treatment

Symptom	Possible cause and related nutritional treatments
Anxiety	Cause: adrenal stress high. Vitamin C, B complex, K, Mg (magnesium), ashwaganda, Zen, support via relaxation and nutrients to support adrenal function
Allergies	Cause: low sulphation. Use cysteine, molybdenum, sulphate, increase essential fatty acids, vitamin C, check for hypothyroidism and eliminate food allergies
Always ill	Use vitamins C, A, E, B$_6$, zinc, selenium, antioxidants, Echinacea, bee propolis, Co-Q10, EFAs to support and strengthen the immune system
Asthma	Take out food allergies and increase vitamin C, vitamin E, flaxseed, magnesium and adrenal support. Modulate the immune system by reducing a Th2 dominance with mycocyclin
Constipation/ diarrhoea	Causes: dysbiosis, low serotonin, low fibre, low water, low magnesium and vitamin C, little exercise. For constipation, decrease insoluble fibre, give high doses of vitamin C, cascara or senna and Oxypowder. Increase water consumption and hydration, provide probiotics, avoid food allergies such as wheat and dairy, support with slippery elm, FOS
Craves foods	Look for food allergies, *Candida*, dysbiosis, blood sugar problems, casein and dairy. If these are problematic, seek advice from your practitioner to help eliminate them

Chart continues on pages 276–278

Symptom	Possible cause and related nutritional treatments
Dark eye circles	Causes: allergies or liver stress. Avoid allergenic foods, support liver function (milk thistle/burdock, increase antioxidants especially glutathione)
Dry/coarse hair	Causes: deficiencies in essential fatty acids and B complex vitamins. Supplement biotin and B vitamins, EFAs, silica. Reduce salt, sugar and refined food
Eczema	Check for food allergies and chemical sensitivities, such as washing powder; use eco balls or soapnuts. Use evening primrose oil, zinc, vitamin E cream, biotin, Mg/Ca (calcium), aloe vera gel, probiotics, omega-3 fish oils
Fatigue	Causes: poor blood sugar balance, low B vitamins, candidiasis, low Mg. Supplement B and Mg, protein with each meal, chromium, check for *Candida*
Hyperactive/ overactive	Causes: excitotoxins and MSG, etc., phenols, sugar, allergies, inflammation, ammonia (arginine), heavy metals. For adrenal stress use Ca/Mg, BCAA (branch chain amino acids), antioxidants, iron, folate, zinc, vitamin B_6, carnitine, vitamins C and B complex, and potassium
Insomnia	Cause: inflammation is very common as this prevents adequate production of serotonin, which then goes on to make melatonin. Use 5HTP, serotonin, melatonin, B_2, B_3, B_6, A, D, folic acid, Ca/Mg, K
Itching and fidgeting	Causes: *Candida*, worms, anxiety, ammonia (sore anal area). Check for all and support their treatment via a qualified practitioner
Mood swings, irritability, and temper tantrums	Causes: heavy metal toxicity, low levels of serotonin commonly due to inflammation, blood sugar imbalances and adrenal stress, plus reactions to food allergens and chemicals, preservatives found within them. Use B_1, B_5, B_6, B_{12}, C, folic acid, Ca/Mg, K, iron, zinc, chromium, iodine

Symptom	Possible cause and related nutritional treatments
Muscle loss	Causes: poor exercise levels or deficiencies in BCAAs, which are isoleucine, leucine, valine
No language/ speech	Causes: common inflammation in the frontal lobe, opioid activity and common deficiencies in omega-3, MB 12*, carnosine, zinc, DMG, acetyl-l-carnitine
PICA (Chewing strange objects)	Iron, zinc, B₆, Mg, Ca and vitamin D. Pica causes sufferers to eat strange non-food items such as chewing rubber balls, stones, sand, grit, soil, collars or cuffs on shirts, laundry soap, buttons, etc.
Picky eater	Cause: driven by food allergies and/or zinc deficiency and sensitivities to colour and texture due to adrenal stress
Rocking	Causes: ear inflammation/anxiety/adrenal stress. Seek advice to identify and treat accordingly
Seizures	Causes: gut toxicity and neurotransmitter imbalances. B₆ and taurine can be supportive
Self-stimulatory behaviour	Causes: low serotonin, streptococcal or Clostridia infection. Identify and treat with 5HTP, omega-3, vitamin C
Sensitivities to texture, tastes and smells	Causes: zinc deficiencies, adrenal stress
General back-up	Vitamins A, C, E, D, B₆, B₁₂, B complex Minerals and trace elements – zinc, magnesium, calcium, selenium, chromium, molybdenum Amino acids: taurine, arginine, lysine, methionine, glycine, cysteine, BCAAs (leucine, isoleucine and valine) Essential fatty acids (EPA/DHA)

*MB 12: Methylcobalamin, a type of B_{12} vitamin.

Gastrointestinal support	Pro- and prebiotics, anti-fungals, anti-microbials, butyrate and glutamine, digestive enzymes, secretin, CCK, 1–3 beta glucans, oxypowder, charcoal, pectin, psyllium, flaxseeds and oil, aloe vera
Detoxification	Increase glutathione by supporting the methylation and transulphation pathway:
	Methylation support: methionine, folinic acid, B_{12} (spray or IV), SAMe, TMG, MSM, B_6, magnesium
	Transulphation support: N-acetyl cysteine (*not* with candidiasis), molybdenum, alpha-lipoic acid, vitamin C, vitamin E, TD glutathione, liposomal glutathione, glycine
	Reduce exposure to food and environmental toxins as these will exhaust antioxidant reserves, especially glutathione and vitamins C, A and E
Heavy-metal elimination via clathration, immune system support and modulation	Nano detox factor, PCA-Rx, lipoic acid, chlorella, cilantro (chelation agents), selenium, zinc. Colostrum, green lipid mussel extract, *Saccharomyces boulaardii*, 1–3, 1–6 beta glucans, mycocyclin, transferfactor, phytocort, lauricidin, antimicrobials such as uva ursi, aged garlic, capryllic acid, berberine, vitamins C, A, E, zinc. Antioxidants pygnenenol, quercetin, bioflavonoids
Reduce inflammation	Remove allergens, kill pathogens
	Omega-3 essential fatty acids especially DHA and EPA
	Antioxidants such as vitamins C, E, A, K, glutathione, cysteine, alpha lipoic acid
	Curcumin, boswelia, pycnogenol, green tea, nettles, slippery elm, cat's claw, di-glycerised liquorice, aloe vera, grape seed extract, N-acetyl cysteine, glucosamine

Remember: all 'symptoms' have a cause! *All* of the symptoms above have an underlying cause and *can* be treated.

Index